The Fit Mum

Formula

The Complete Diet & Lifestyle Plan created exclusively for Mums
by Pollyanna Hale

www.thefitmumformula.com

First Published in Great Britain in 2016

Copyright © 2016 Pollyanna Hale

ISBN: 978-0-9929731-6-2 (pbk)
         978-0-9929731-7-9 (ebk)

Design by The Fit Mum Formula Ltd.

Production Shakspeare Editorial

CONTENTS

YOUR FREE GIFT!

How would you like to have convenient, portable and delicious complete meals ready in 5 minutes?!

As a thank you bonus for buying this book I'm sending you a free copy of my ebook *How To Make A Supershake*

To receive your ebook, leave a review on Amazon, take a screenshot and a screenshot of your order confirmation, and email them to me at polly@thefitmumformula.com

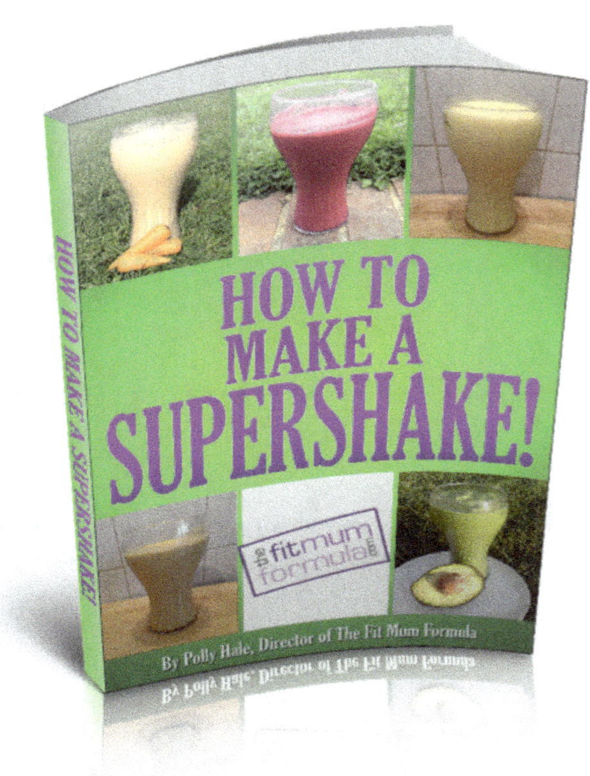

Acknowledgements

This book would not exist without business coach Anthony Deximer. Not because he's my coach, or because he had a hand in its creation (in three months from start to finish), but it was in a simple Skype call with him that he managed to persuade me I did in fact have the time, if I chose to. Not any easy persuasion, as a Mum of two young girls, as well as running The Fit Mum Formula, it's not like I'm not pushing the boundaries of my time already. But what can I say? An hour a day before the girls get up for school and here you are reading it.

My website developers Liam Thompson and Matt Murphy and tech/Facebook advert extraordinaire Aimee Holland. Thanks for putting up with my endless bimbo support tickets.

Alison Shakspeare, the most loyal editor and expert on all things books and writing.

James, Bella and Aurora, you didn't really see this book being written as for the most part you were all still asleep in bed. Thank you for the silence, and for putting up with a tired and grumpy wife/Mum occasionally, and for all the pictures, cards and cuddles. I love them even when you don't put the pens away.

My up and coming fitpro sister Mel, the only person in my family I can 'talk shop' with when we choose to, while everyone discusses politics/how to cook a turkey/best scene in Paw Patrol.

My cafetiere, you might need a new plunger and leak ground coffee into my cup, but our morning meetings have been integral to the completion of this book, and accompanying marketing that I battled to get set up, as all the support tickets (see above) show.

And to everyone who got the free chapter, pre-ordered or bought the final book, I wrote it for you, it means a lot that you value it and saw the value in it for yourself. I won't give up on you if you won't.

INTRODUCTION

LET'S GET TO KNOW EACH OTHER

You are most likely reading this book because you are looking to do one or more of the following things:

- have more energy

- burn fat

- tone up

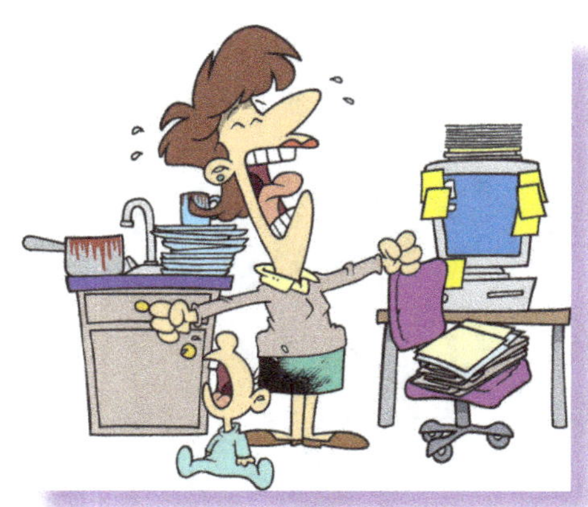

I'm a busy Mum just like you. I'm also just like every other woman in that I really do want to take pride in myself, look after my body, feel good about the way I look and have loads of energy. But with two small children (at the time of writing Aurora is seven, so now in School, Bella is four and still at home with me, except for three mornings at Nursery), plus a home to run and husband to cook for and clean up after; that leaves very little time and energy left for us Mums to have 'me time'.

Child-free time for the gym or classes? Nope.

Strict meal plans than mean making separate meals for everyone? No thank you.

An hour a day to exercise? If only!

I used to be at a full-time Performing Arts school, and dancing 5–7 hours a day kept me extremely fit. But by the time I switched to do a Health and Beauty Therapy Management qualification I was fed up of pushing my body to extremes, so stopped exercising altogether and instead kept my weight low on a diet of processed food, low calorie junk food snacks, like fat-free cookies and diet ice cream, while staying on my feet all day as a beauty therapist.

And that's where it spiralled downwards …

I nearly died of an eating disorder

I'VE GOT TO WARN YOU THIS IS RAW

I love food, especially food that makes you feel good. But I wasn't always like this, not by a long way. In fact, I nearly died.

It took me 10 years to 'come out' and open up to the world, many of whom never knew anything about it. People I saw every day didn't even know.

But it's important for me to be honest with you, and to be true to myself. I'm hoping it will help other people just knowing they're not alone.

Why am I so passionate about health? Because I nearly died. I was extremely ill with anorexia for a few years. I was a dangerously low weight, my organs were failing, and I was in and out of psychiatric hospitals for years, once even sectioned under the Mental Health Act.

Against all odds I recovered, and now nourish and strengthen my body to be the best it can be. The words 'strong not skinny' are my mantra for the way I eat and exercise.

I now coach other women to get the body and the body confidence they want with online coaching. Most women come to me wanting to lose weight not gain it. But it doesn't matter as it's all the same really – caring for your body and treating it well so that it becomes the body you deserve.

I hope you won't judge me. I hope instead you will see that I'm not perfect but I have learnt a LOT, and I hope I can pass this wisdom on to you.

You only have one body, look after it.

What doesn't kill you makes you stronger, literally.

My coming out video can be viewed here, though I warn you, if you've had mental health problems yourself it could be triggering:

https://www.facebook.com/thefitmumformula/videos/1141103185941354/

Then I made a video to try and inspire others to break away from their limiting thoughts and behaviours and show them that loving and caring for your body is possible.

My *Strong Not Skinny* video can be viewed here:

https://www.facebook.com/thefitmumformula/videos/1196484663736539/

After recovery

My weight and mental health stabilised but I wasn't the person I am today. I was very slim, but I wasn't fit or strong. I was a classic 'skinny fat'. I had no energy, slept poorly and, though I fitted into size 6 clothes, in a bikini my body looked like one of someone much older – I had absolutely no muscle tone, and once I had my first daughter in 2009, well, as you can imagine, I had real problems with my tummy and back after carrying a 7 lb 11 oz baby (I'm only 5 ft. 2). At one time I even looked into surgery to get my 'abs' back together because I'd heard a rumour that's what Madonna did! Yet, with a baby to look after at home I had even less time to devote to my own health.

But all that changed when I was introduced to some concepts that changed my life, attitudes toward my health and my body. The idea that to get my body, health and energy back I need to fuel it properly and build muscle, while at the same time burning fat (remember I said I was 'skinny fat'? Yes, I had fat over the top of those bones!).

It's not always as simple as eating fewer calories and moving around more. That's what got me into that mess in the first place!

So I read every book I could get my hands on, tried and tested exercise techniques, investigated various dietary methods, and qualified as a Personal Trainer (PT) specialising in circuits and kettlebell training. I became a Metabolic Conditioning Nutritional Consultant and was granted a certificate by the Association For Nutrition – all the while working on myself and with other women to learn the techniques that are best for females who need to lose weight and tone up while having more energy, but need results fast with minimal time and effort put in.

With hardly any time or energy to exercise and plan laborious meals I had to think of a way for Mums to get their pre-baby body back with techniques that required minimum time and effort. The information had to be delivered in a way that revolves around family life, so an online programme is the only option for most Mums. The Fit Mum Formula was born.

ARE DIETS EFFECTIVE? LET'S LOOK BACK AT YOUR DIETING HISTORY

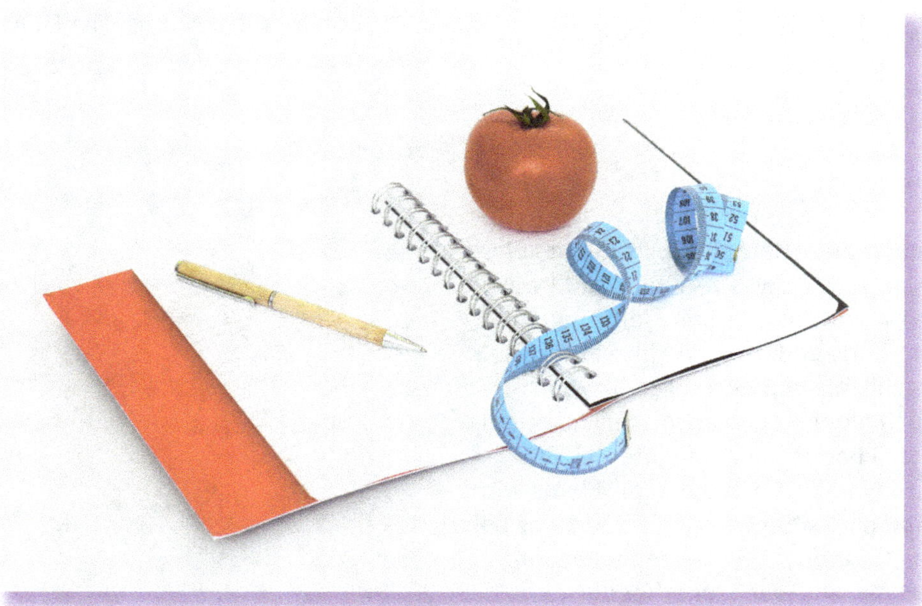

It's a sorry fact that today more people in developed countries are either overweight and/or dieting than those who aren't. Being on a diet is so common that we are actually surprised when we meet someone who 'just eats normally'!

Fads and trends come and go, usually accompanied by celebrity endorsements and a wonderful array of marketing tactics, but do today's popular diet plans actually work?

There's a thought that if diets worked, none of us would ever need to be on one. So maybe that's the problem – it's not the diet itself that's holding us back, but our ability to stick with them.

What makes a good diet long term? Well, as well as keeping you feeling, looking and performing at your best – whatever that means to you – it has to fit into your lifestyle in a convenient and not too disruptive way. You have to enjoy it. And it has to have enough room for manoeuvre to adapt to whatever is going on in your life and wherever you are.

But many people resort to temporary diets to kick-start their weight loss, which is fine if it is indeed temporary, which means knowing how to continue eating healthily once you reach your goal weight or come to end of the 'plan'. Unfortunately, that's where short-term diets fall down – they don't teach long-term habits and strategies for health.

Five of the most popular diets and why they may or may not work for you

Which of these have you tried in the past?

LOW CARB

Reduced consumption of starchy carbohydrates like rice, potatoes and pasta, and often dairy and fruit, which also contain carbohydrates. Going really low carb also means restricting the amount of higher carb vegetables consumed, such as beetroot, carrots and squash, and sticking to mostly lean proteins and green vegetables. It is thought that reducing carbohydrates helps to balance blood sugar and therefore energy levels, as well as keeping hunger to a minimum (protein and veg are really filling).

Pros

Very filling without over-consuming calories. Restricted food choices make meal planning easier – the guidelines and options are clear and simple; just cut out the starchy part.

Cons

Going too low carb doesn't work for everyone, and some people don't feel great without enough carbs to suit their own physiology. Though you can make and buy low carb treats, traditional sugary snacks are off limits, which can, in some people, lead to binges later down the line when they feel too restricted.

PALEO

Eating 'ancestrally' is not meant in the literal sense, in that many of the meat and vegetables around thousands of years ago don't even exist anymore, and, in addition, it's still Paleo to eat modern foods created from paleo ingredients, like nut based cookies or avocado 'cheesecake'. All grains and dairy are cut out, as well as legumes, alcohol and, of course, processed foods of any sort, including most sugars except a honey or other similar natural sugars.

Pros

No processed foods and only whole, natural, nutrient-dense foods makes this an extremely nutritious way of eating that will almost certainly be providing you with all the vitamins, minerals and other nutrients you need to feel and perform at your best. Cutting out dairy and gluten in particular (two of the most 'problematic' foods) can also increase energy and decrease digestive and other problems in many people.

Cons

While most Paleo followers eat relatively low carb, this isn't an essential requisite, nor is calorie counting, and so, while the types of food eaten are restricted (and very nutritious), overall quantity and proportions of fat, carbohydrate and protein guidelines are vague, which means you won't necessarily be getting the right balance of macronutrients for you. It's also very easy to over or under eat if you're not being mindful of energy intake. There are health benefits to all of the banned foods like dairy, so if you don't have an issue digesting these, you may be cutting them out unnecessarily.

5:2 DIET

A form of intermittent fasting, on two days a week only 500/600 calories (for women or men respectively) are consumed, while a 'normal' diet of 2,000/2,400 calories are eaten on the other five days. This results in an overall calorie deficit over the week and therefore weight loss, as well as other purported health benefits, such as improved blood pressure and cholesterol profile, and improved insulin sensitivity – leading to improvements in diabetes or reduced chances of developing the disease.

Pros

Learning to go for longer without eating and being able to live with hunger are skills that, in the long run, will mean you feel less inclined to snack at the first tummy rumble. Cutting calories drastically will result in an overall reduction in calories over the week – as long as you don't make up for it by over-consuming on non-fast days – so weight loss is a likely outcome. It may improve insulin sensitivity in some people and reduce the chances of developing diabetes.

Cons

500 calories in a day is not very much at all and many people will struggle with hunger, low energy and poor concentration. Women tend to fare worse with intermittent fasting as our hormones stay better balanced when we don't go too long without eating, and not everyone has improved insulin sensitivity and are better off sticking to a more consistent eating pattern.

MEAL REPLACEMENT PLANS

Slim Fast, Lighter Life, Cambridge ... You don't have to have cooking skills, or indeed any nutritional knowledge at all, when your meals consist of ready-made bars, shakes, soups and sometimes microwave meals. All products are calorie restricted, which means that if you stick to the plan and eat only the products provided almost everyone will lose weight simply because they're consuming fewer calories than they're burning.

Pros

Convenient, time saving and no cooking/preparing/calorie counting required. Available at most supermarkets and some health food stores and chemists.

Cons

Pre-made foods will never match up nutritionally to fresh, whole, natural foods, especially when many of these products use cheap ingredients and bulking agents. Adding vitamins and minerals to the ingredients will make no difference if the added nutrients are not of the highest quality (which would make the end product much more expensive than they already are), as our bodies just don't absorb these synthetic nutrients well. Taste is obviously subjective, but sticking to the same products day in day out may result in flavour fatigue, where you get so sick and bored of eating the same things you are more likely to go off track and not stick to the plan.

VEGAN

There's only one rule on a vegan diet, and that's that nothing consumed can be of animal origin. Meals comprise vegetables, fruit, legumes, soy, grains, nuts and seeds. Meat or fish, eggs and dairy are not allowed, and neither is the gelatine used in commercial sweets and puddings. Most people who eat a vegan diet do so for health rather than weight loss, and with no parameters for macronutrients (protein, carbohydrates and fat) or calorie intake, health and weight outcomes are very much dependent on an individual's food intake. Vegans tend to be health conscious by nature and often consume lots of whole, natural foods, with lots of vegetables and fruit, though this isn't a requisite of a vegan diet.

Pros

If tonnes of vegetables, fruit, high fibre legumes and some grains are consumed then this way of eating can be very nutritious. Vitamin and fibre intake is undoubtedly high, and it's likely that no or minimal processed foods are consumed, as most processed foods contain animal products of some sort.

Cons

It's very hard to get all the nutrients you need without consuming meat and fish, or eggs and dairy. The same nutrients that are in these foods – such as calcium, iron, and omega-3 fats – just aren't absorbed as well from plant sources. Vitamin B12, which is needed for energy, is only found in animal foods, so all vegans should be supplementing with this vitamin at the very least.

So, are popular diets worth the hype? Do they work?

I think the answer is both yes and no. Any diet will 'work' if you follow it in the right way for your goals, for long enough. Ultimately though you need be asking yourself, is this way of eating contributing to my health? Or taking away from it?

In the next section we'll take a look at the how our eating patterns have changed over time, and how our bodies have changed with it.

THE DEMISE OF OUR DIET

You'd think that time brings wisdom, but looking at the eating habits of the Western world, the contents of our cupboards, the restaurants and fast food chains we go to, it appears not.

For the first 190,000 of our 200,000 or so years on the planet humans were hunter gatherers. We ate when we could get food; sometimes this was a lot, but other times there was no food for days. We ate meat (the whole animal, not just muscle meat), fish, tubers (root vegetables), plants and vegetables and fruits where available and in season, nuts, insects, and anything else we could get our hands on that wouldn't poison us (likely through lots of sad-ending trial and error). Exactly what we ate would have depended on the time of year (seasonality) and where we lived (what grew there). So there is no one 'Palaeolithic diet', just a selection of foods that were available in certain parts of the world, some of the time.

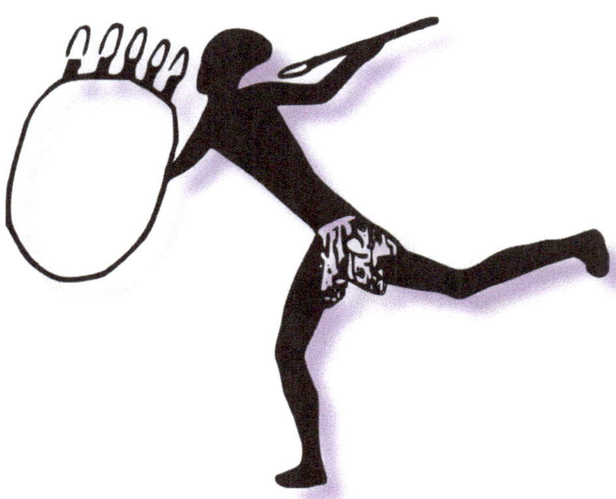

Humans were highly active – walking and hunting, climbing, gathering and carrying. They were likely fit and strong. The average life of Palaeolithic man was low but, contrary to what we first thought about this being due to their basic and unevolved life, it was much more likely due to being caught by prey, or being injured and having no means of medical care, leading to lethal infections, or being left to die by other tribe members – a person with a severely broken leg that can't be fixed is a serious burden on a tribe.

What we do know from studies is that obesity, heart disease, diabetes and other 'modern'

diseases were rare, so if you, by pure chance, didn't get eaten or broken, people would have lived a long and healthy life.

Harvard University's evolutionary biologist Daniel Lieberman believes that, "Many of the illnesses that we confront today are what evolutionary biologists called 'mismatch diseases': ... Diseases that occur because our bodies are poorly or inadequately adapted to environments in which we now live. An example would be eating large amounts of sugar or being very physically inactive leads to problems like diabetes or heart disease that then make us sick."

In other words, our bodies are not responding well to our current lifestyle choices, not just with food but also our activity levels, hygiene habits and stress levels. That's why diseases such as diabetes and heart disease, mental illnesses such as depression – and some people even include cancer – are coined 'lifestyle diseases', as opposed to say, contagious diseases like malaria or diphtheria.

The health timeline

Note that for years, dates and facts weren't recorded nearly as rigorously as we do today, the dates here are estimates based on the few records found and studies done.

- around 20,000 BC – humans gathered grains when and where they grew, and ate them any way that was palatable and digestible, either whole or ground. The types of grains that grew are rarely, if ever, grown on earth today, at least for commercial use

- 10,000 BC – grains began to be cultivated in the Middle East, Eastern Europe and parts of Africa. These included emmer and einkorn wheat, hulled barley, peas, lentils, bitter vetch, chickpeas and flax

- 1600s – start of the British Agricultural Revolution, when commercial grain productivity became among the highest in the world

- 1900s – large rises in productivity as human labour was replaced by mechanization, and assisted by synthetic fertilizers, pesticides and selective breeding; vegetable oils are introduced into foods and households; trans fats are invented; flours become stripped and milled; and sugar becomes widely available as travel and importation increases

- 1970s – high fructose corn syrup is introduced

- 1983 – low fat diet recommendations were introduced, encouraging high carbohydrate consumption in place of fat

- 2007 – the UK 'Eatwell Plate' is introduced, advising people on the different proportions of each food group to eat. This is in line with the low fat, high carbohydrate advice of the 1980s.

- 2016 – the US Dietary Guidelines are revised, removing the advice to avoid dietary cholesterol from foods such as eggs, after no link was found to heart disease; the advice to eat a high carb, low fat diet still stands.

What effect have these changes had on us?

- incidents of diabetes have increased 59.9% since 2005

- since 1890 childhood obesity rates in the US (the UK are not far behind) have tripled; 17.7% of 6–11 years olds and 20.5% of teenagers are obese

- by 2005 the total number of cardiovascular disease deaths had increased globally to 17.5 million, up from 14.4 million in 1990

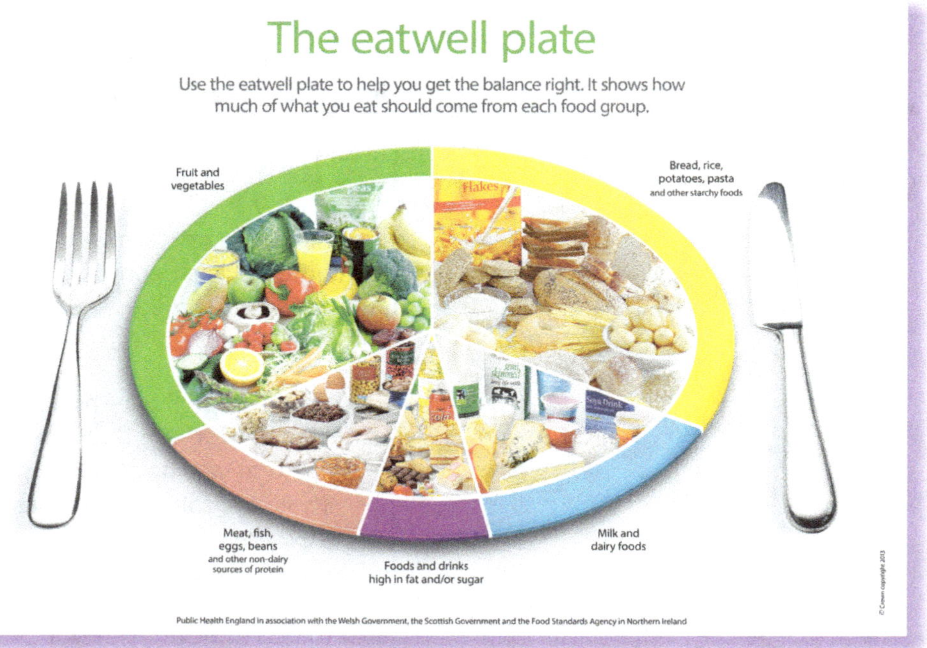

- 2016 – the 'Eatwell Guide' replaces the Eatwell Plate and advice includes an increase in fruit, vegetables and starchy carbohydrates, while sugary treats and drinks are no longer included

- if current trends continue and no action is taken, the number of people with dementia in the UK is forecast to increase to 1,142,677 by 2025 and 2,092,945 by 2051, an increase of 40% over the next 12 years and of 156% over the next 38 years

- in England the prevalence of obesity among adults rose from 14.9% to 25.6% between 1993 and 2014

- the number of people diagnosed in the UK with coeliac disease increased fourfold between 1990 and 2011, a study suggests

- occurrence of mental health issues, such as depression and anxiety, among women aged 45–64 rose by about a 5th between 1993 and 2005

- the prevalence of ADHD drug use in children under 16 has increased 34-fold, rising from 1.5 per 10,000 children in 1995 to 50.7 per 10,000 children in 2008, then stabilising at 51.1 per 10,000 children in 2013

- cancer incidence rates in the UK have increased by 30% since the late 1970s

- agriculturalists are shorter than, and have more cavities, smaller brains and weaker bones than hunter-gatherers, according to researchers at Cambridge University

- by 2050 obesity is predicted to affect 60% of adult men, 50% of adult women and 25% of children

- life expectancy has increased, however, this is more likely due to medical advances and drugs that are able to keep a person alive despite the numerous health issues they carry, than due to better health.

Are we all doomed, then?

Of course, these correlations don't prove that our lifestyle and dietary changes caused the demise of our health, but it certainly is, *ahem*, food for thought. Other changes we've seen that may have contributed include:

- a dramatic increase in pesticide and herbicide use in crop cultivation

- animals we eat being given hormones and antibiotics to maximise growth and/or egg/milk output

- the profligate use of antibiotics to treat minor illnesses (and even viruses, where they are useless)

- more pollution, from cars and factories

- the development and prolific use of chemical cleaning agents

- an increase in chemically based toiletry and cosmetic use

- we are increasingly stressed; we pack more and more into our day and sleep less

- a dramatic decrease in our daily physical activity, not only in transport (we prefer to drive, even short distances), but with the availability of household gadgets, such as washing machines and hedge trimmers, that make light work of physical tasks.

Two points to make here.

1. Dissecting and evaluating all of these is beyond the scope of this book, and there are many knowledgeable professionals far more qualified than I to talk about these subjects.

2. Not in any way am I suggesting you should make your life harder than it has to be by scrubbing your clothes or walking 15 miles a day to fetch some clean water.

What I am suggesting is that the following small steps may (read: likely will) help improve your health and wellbeing:

- use eco-friendly household cleaning products, natural toiletries and cosmetics

- don't use cleaning agents at all where possible; hot water and a good cloth/scrubber will suffice in most cases

- deal with bad smells with a few drops of essential oils; lemon and tea tree oil are great, the latter is also a natural antibacterial

- buy organic food where possible, it doesn't cost as much more as you think, and most people are spending money on things they don't really want, which they could cut out

- sleep, rest and lots to drink will help most minor illnesses cure themselves; being healthy will also boost your immunity dramatically and stop you getting ill in the first place

- consider taking a probiotic; bacteria play a huge role in our health, and most people need more of them in their gut

- counteract any non-flexible sedentary activities (for example, working in an office) with enough physical activity elsewhere in your life

- be realistic about what you can fit into one day; stop setting the bar so high; there is a very important time and place to just do nothing (for the record, I'm really bad at this, but I'm working on it!)

And importantly, and what I encourage for the majority of your diet is:

Just. Eat. Real. Food.

Caveat: there are a great many convenient, shop bought, nutritious foods available (especially in the case of snack foods) that have been made in a factory. Some of these are made with 'real food' but look no different on the packet than ones that market themselves as healthy but are actually pretty non-nutritious. So, just because something comes in a packet, does not inherently make it junk.

The difficulty comes in being able to decipher labels and understand ingredients. Some natural ingredients sound like an artificial additive because you're not familiar with the name. Take *ascorbyl palmitate*; this is an antioxidant made from vitamin C and palmitic acid, a natural compound derived from fat. On the other hand, the (so-called, natural) sweet syrup *agave nectar* is actually highly processed and refined, and very high in fructose, a type of sugar that puts strain on the liver. Yes, fructose is found in fruit, but in much more reasonable amounts in relation to the water, fibre and beneficial vitamins in fresh fruit.

So no, you don't have to start making every meal and snack totally from scratch, 100% of the time (we are busy Mums after all!). Knowing what to look for, and how to create a great (but not perfect) diet is what we're aiming for. Plus, fish fingers are so darn tasty.

Evolution or lifestyle?

Human lives have changed dramatically over the last few thousand years, but our genetics have changed very little.

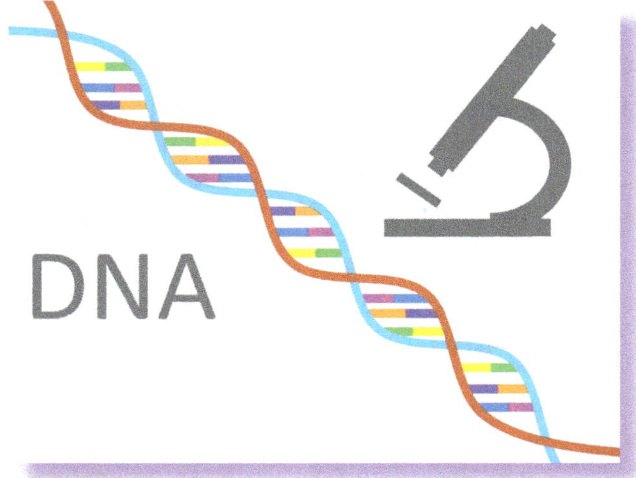

The funny thing is, there are genes for diabetes, cancer, even obesity, but these genes can be switched on or off. This is called 'gene expression'. That means that, whatever set of genetics you were born with, you will only become fat, physically or psychologically ill, if those genes become switched on. Many factors will also come into play, for example, life stressors such as divorce or death might lead to someone becoming depressed. But even then, the result is often more physiological than you think.

When you are stressed, hormones such as cortisol and adrenaline, normally reserved for life-threatening events (such as giving you the reflex and energy to run from a burning building or get out of the way of a car being driven wildly), are released in abnormally large amounts over a long period of time. This has a domino effect across the body, causing trouble everywhere it goes. Leaky gut (also known as gut permeability) means undigested food particles get into your bloodstream leading to intolerances and allergies as your immune system jumps into action. At the same time, the immune system can become supressed, so you get ill more easily. Cortisol elevates blood sugar levels, which puts stress on its natural regulation and can lead to diabetes. Cortisol constricts blood vessels and increases blood pressure to enhance the delivery of oxygenated blood, which is why stressed out people are more at risk of heart disease. Long-term stress and elevated cortisol may also be linked to insomnia, chronic fatigue syndrome, thyroid disorders, dementia, depression and other conditions.

So back to the point, many psychological conditions have a physiological route, and by having a healthy body you become more resilient to the effects that any life stressors might have on your mind and body. It's clear some people are more resilient than others. One example is the eating disorder I had as a teenager. I was at dance school (highly pressured in terms of the way you look) and my parents divorced when I was a child. Two factors that may have influenced any psychological stress. But not everyone whose parents get divorced, or who go to a pressured dance school, end up with an eating disorder. There must have been other factors at play. Perhaps if I'd known better (and to be fair, how could I?), I could have built a stronger, healthier body that was more equipped to deal with any stress or trauma that came my way.

What about you, have you ever experienced prolonged stress, depression, anxiety, maybe binge eating? Have you ever wondered whether you might not have developed these conditions had your body been in a better place, physically, at the time? I won't go off at too much of a tangent here, but much research is happening as we speak as to how dietary interventions, gut healing and bacteria levels (the 'microbiome') can play a huge role in treating everything from depression, to ADHD, to Alzheimer's to Autism. I, personally, can't wait to see this approach become more mainstream.

I'm not a doctor or a scientist, and I personally don't think I'll be able to change our entire nation's approach to health by myself. But when tired, stressed out, overweight but undernourished and desperate Mums come to me for help, I'm going to over deliver. Because, while you think you've come to me to lose weight and improve your fitness and energy levels – though that's likely true and I will show you how to do that – by following the advice in this book you will be getting so much more than that.

You'll be happier, less stressed, have less brain fog and better focus and concentration. You'll get ill less often, recover faster when you do, and be able to handle more responsibilities in less time.

That's not to say I expect you to be perfect all of the time. That's a) not possible, and b) not realistic. In fact, I'd argue that anyone who is a strict 'perfectionist', to the point where everything is always done perfectly, has some issues that are preventing them from accepting themselves just as they are. Perfectionism was a big part of my anorexia, and accepting ourselves as imperfect is essential for happiness.

In this book I'll be sharing with you my Formula that creates a happy body and mind, and in following it you'll learn just how good it is possible to look and feel about your body. As my personal story shows, you can be slim but that won't make you happy. Both matter for long-term success, health and happiness.

And it all starts with setting your goals correctly, which I'll cover in the next section.

WHY MUMS ARE NOT YOUR AVERAGE CLIENT

Any half decent PT knows how to create a plan that results in weight loss for new Mums (or anyone for that matter), with the right choice and quantity of exercise combined with a calorie deficit of nutritionally dense foods in the right proportions.

Likewise, for post-natal specialists who deal with diastasis recti (where the abdominal muscles don't close correctly following pregnancy) and pelvic floor issues; with the right education you have the knowledge to help your clients. Heck, you don't have to be a parent (or even a female trainer) to devise a programme for a women to get back to her old self (or as close as reasonable) after becoming a Mummy.

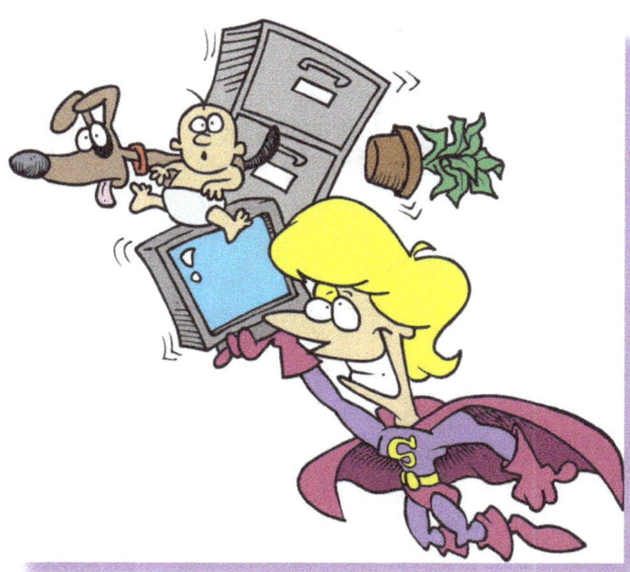

I'm talking about the details that are hard to envisage unless you're actually a parent yourself, or unless you spend a significant amount of time regularly with other parents.

The saying goes that nothing can prepare you for being a parent or for the challenges of parenthood. As the eldest child of eight kids and with my youngest sister being 15 years my junior, I've never been blind to what it takes to look after small people. But having my own? My own body being challenged to grow another person, feed another person (I breastfed both my daughters for two years +), being responsible for their every need – BTW this last bit doesn't really reduce as they get older, the responsibilities just move on from

helping to expel wind, to nose wiping, to helping backstage at ballet recitals, and so it goes on.

Motherhood (parenthood, I don't want to exclude Dads here, though statistically it is most likely to be the Mums who are the predominant child carers) is the most amazing feat in the world, but it's a round the clock job with no holidays, no sick pay, not even time off for sickness, and many challenges along the way that prove to be hurdles that slow a mother's progress from carrying 'baby-weight' to shedding said baby-weight.

Here's a rundown of some of the reasons for struggling to get in shape that are exclusive to parents.

WE ARE SLEEP DEPRIVED AND IT'S NOT OUR FAULT

Even if your darling slept through the night from 3 months old (darn I envy you), there will inevitably be times – night potty training, illness, nightmares, Christmas morning (hello over-excited kids at 4am!) – when you won't get enough sleep.

Sleep is critical for all bodily functions including growing and maintaining muscle mass, burning fat, exercise recovery and appetite management. No athlete at the top of their game, either sporting performance or aesthetic (in the case of stage competitions or modelling), will succeed without making sleep a priority. Try telling that to a two-year-old who has decided that sleeping is not on the agenda tonight. So it stands to reason that a sleep deprived parent will struggle in all these areas.

What can help?

You can't stop it, but you can help manage symptoms. Epsom salts in baths are wonderful for less-than recovered aching muscles. Relaxing essential oils on a pillow may help make the sleep a parent gets at least of the good quality, deep kind, even if quantity can't be achieved. Emphasising protein, fibre, and quality fats in the diet will help manage hunger. Green tea (or even black tea) is a low calorie pick me up that also contains L-Theanine, an amino acid that is highly relaxing, and the caffeine (note – avoid drinking in excess or near bedtime) can actually be an appetite suppressant in some people too. Green tea contains EGCG which has been shown to boost the metabolism, burning fat and providing you with energy at the same time.

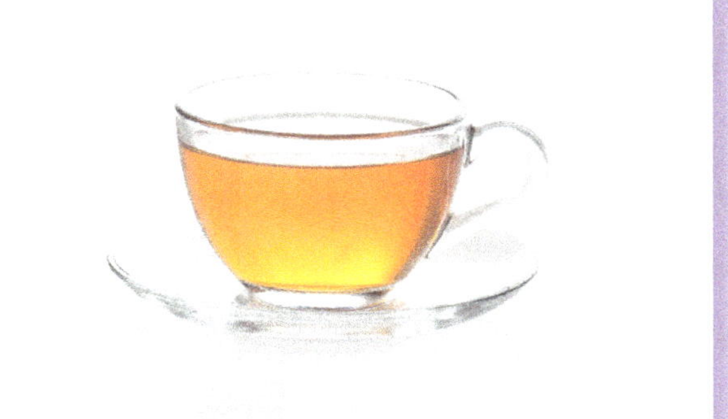

PARENTS ARE VERY STRESSED

People often assume stress is of the 'bad' kind – financial problems, fights with a loved one, huge workloads, illness and relationship issues – but parents are some of the happiest yet most stressed people of all. Anything which taxes the body and/ or brain is stressful – lack of sleep, poor food, alcohol, exercise, even just having a lot of things to remember (sports kit, book bag, Disney character lunch box, gloves …). Do not underestimate the power of stress. It is linked to so many medical issues, from cardiovascular disease to diabetes, to obesity, to IBS … the list goes on.

From a 'getting in shape' perspective it lowers our cognitive abilities to make good (healthy) decisions. It also drives people to comfort eat, even without realising they're doing it, or alternatively to lose their appetite and not eat.

What can help?

These things take practice and consistency to make them habits, but they take no time, no equipment and can be done anywhere, which makes them non-negotiable for pretty much everyone, parent or not.

1. Deep breathing: take three slow, deep breaths, allowing the air to go deep into your belly – it is the belly not the chest that needs to expand – any time you feel stressed.

2. Lower your shoulders down and back. Elongate your neck. Correcting this will take time as the muscles that are keeping shoulders raised may be shortened, but like any muscle in the body these too can be retrained and lengthened to stay down and relaxed.

3. Get into nature: 5 minutes with a cup of tea in the garden, 10 minutes picking up conkers with the kids in autumn, 15 minutes making daisy chains. Being among greenery has been shown to lower stress levels, likewise a leisurely walk. If you walk to school or work, leave a little earlier so you can take your time and admire your surroundings.

4. Avoid decision fatigue and don't have too many options, so decision making is easier. Schedule and plan what you're going to eat, what you'll do for exercise and when, and just do that. The decision has been made in advance, all you have to do is follow the plan. If 'rules' make decision making easier, they can help so long as they are in line with your goals and needs. A vegetarian doesn't eat meat because it fits with their values and 'rules'. Having your own 'rules', like only eating cake on weekends or having at least one green vegetable with every evening meal, can take at least some of the decision making (and therefore stress) away.

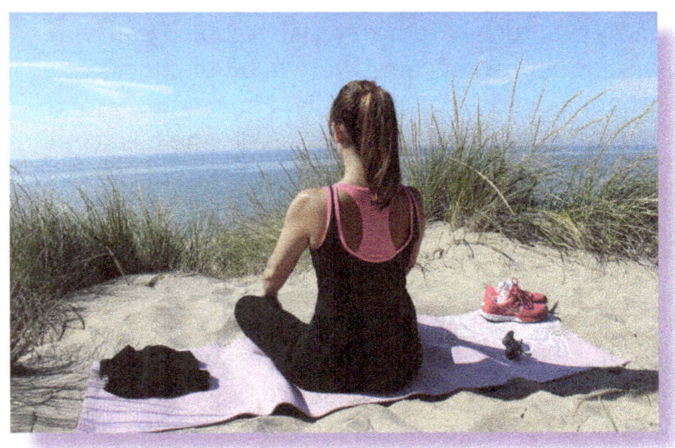

WE HAVE ACCESS TO KIDS' LEFTOVER FOOD

Food costs money, takes time and effort to prepare. Children don't always finish their plate of food, and well done to them – they're in touch with their appetite and stop when they are full. We also know that waste is costly – waste not want not and all that. And their food is tasty, and hopefully good quality most of the time too. But if you're nibbling constantly on what's left on their plates it contributes to excess calories, and this will slow, halt, or even reverse weight loss.

What can help?

If your kids always leave food then this might sound obvious, but you're probably giving them too much. You have two options, either make less, or make more so there's enough to have again another day. I find my kids get 'bored' quickly, so it's better to give them a not oversized main meal then allow them a healthy pudding (fruit, yoghurt, etc.).

Another trick I like is to actually factor those leftovers into your daily intake – provided the food they are being given is nutritious. I could think of worse late afternoon snacks than a fish finger and some peas, just have that instead of, rather than as well as, another snack you make for yourself. Or have a smaller evening meal. It can all be made to add up right in the end.

WE ARE NEAR OUR CUPBOARDS (THAT ARE FULL OF FOOD)

Having to go from desk to canteen/vending machine takes money and effort and is a deterrent, however small, to purchasing that iced bun mid-afternoon. Stay at home parents are within a few feet of food most of the day. This convenience makes it much harder to resist grabbing half a biscuit here, a few nuts there, a bit of chocolate from an ever-shrinking bar. Not having tasty food in the house is not an option. Everyone has to eat, even 'treats' sometimes, and multiple food shopping trips a week are impractical.

What can help?

Set an eating schedule; certain times of the day for meals and snacks. Then don't eat when it isn't 'time'. This schedule has to be sufficient to cover your hunger and needs; there's no point in attempting only three 'traditionally timed' meals a day if you're ravenous with low blood sugar at 4pm every day. It also has to be flexible; eating times can move earlier or later according to what you're doing that day, but sticking to some sort of structure will help curb mindless grazing all day.

If you must 'pick' at food, make sure there's something readily available that will make little

contribution to your daily calories. Fresh berries are one of my favourites for this – low sugar, low calorie, nutrient dense, and little enough to 'pick at' every so often.

And finally, if you are genuinely hungry or have blood sugar problems, consider what you're actually eating at meal times. A balanced meal with enough protein, fibre, fat and carbohydrates to suit your needs should not leave you hungry or needing more food soon afterwards.

WE CAN'T GET TO THE GYM OR EXERCISE CLASSES

Even if our local establishment has a crèche, who's to say I'm happy putting my small child in a room of strangers who, even if adequately qualified and capable, are unfamiliar to my little one, who resents being left without understanding why (no dig at Mums who make use of crèche facilities, it just isn't for me or my kids). Childcare is an added cost, is not always available, and not always preferable for some parents.

What can help?

Newsflash: you don't have to go out to exercise! I developed The Fit Mum Formula for this very reason, to give women access to the knowledge and resources they need to get in shape from home. With a few key exercises, you need minimal space, no equipment, and with enough intensity (such as HIIT workouts) you can get a really good workout done in under 20 minutes. My favourites? Push ups, burpees, squat and lunge variations and bicycle crunches. Add a pair of dumb-bells into the mix and the options are innumerable.

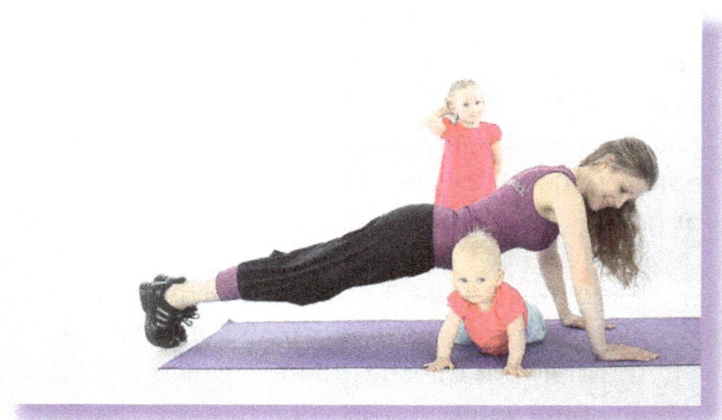

WE ARE SURROUNDED BY CAKE

I've never been to a parent and toddler group that didn't offer tea and cake. I witness on a weekly basis Mums who declare they deserve that homemade brownie with fudge icing because they lost another pound at [insert popular weight loss club here]. The same women are going to the same club when they're attending school plays and parent-teacher evenings.

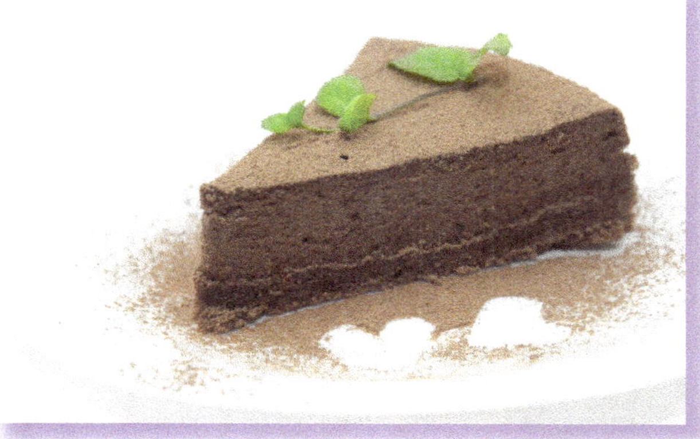

What can help?

Take a snack with you, a piece of fruit, a healthy (as in really healthy, not the 'pretend but actually processed and full of sugar healthy') snack bar, etc. Then you can eat when everyone else does.

Another option? Make this a weekly treat. But mind that it has to be *in place of* other high calorie treats not *as well as*. Some people prefer weekends as the time to have that ice cream/pudding/cake, so you have to make that decision.

OUR HORMONES ARE ALL OVER THE PLACE

OK, 'all over the place' is not the most scientific term, but I don't claim to be an expert on female hormones. It's safe to say, however, that with pregnancy, birth, breastfeeding, the eventual return to menstruation and all of the hormone changes that happen along the way, it can feel like your body and brain are a little unpredictable at best, utter chaos at worst, and that's not even counting things like the aforementioned sleep deprivation. To say breastfeeding burns calories is to dismiss the whole picture. Some women find burning fat while nursing near impossible, while others can't eat enough to keep the weight on and milk supply up. Some women balloon during pregnancy with

minimal changes to their eating habits, others don't put on much weight at all, yet are constantly eating. Don't blame 'eating [cake] for two' as the problem in every case.

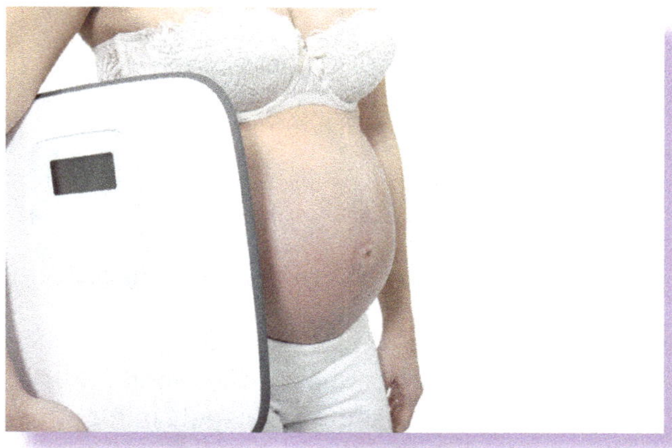

What can help?

Unfortunately this is part of the biological process that is becoming a mother, but luckily most women's bodies do return to a more balanced 'normal', whatever that means to them. Keeping a diary of how you feel mentally and physically might show up patterns to make life more predictable – if baby is going through a growth spurt and feeding more are you more hungry or tired? Or are you noticing any changes as you cut down breastfeeding (or if you didn't breastfeed then a few weeks post birth) that make you think your periods could be making a return soon? How do these changes affect your eating and exercise habits?

It's truly wonderful being a Mum and I wouldn't have it any other way. It's also challenging, exhausting and all consuming. As a fitness, nutrition and weight loss coach I play a part in helping Mums get back some of their energy, vitality and sense of self. Everyone benefits when the right support and strategies are in place. After all, a healthy and happy Mum brings up healthy and happy kids.

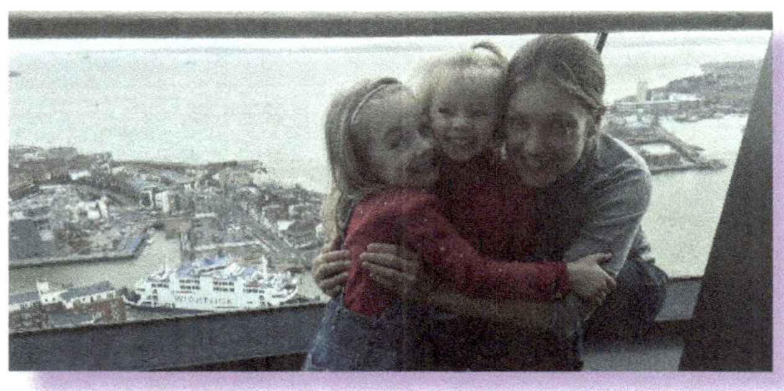

How it works

There are three ways you can get more energy:

1. Eat foods high in starches and sugar. When you eat these foods, sugar enters your bloodstream, and some of this gets burnt as energy. Some of that sugar is removed from your blood by insulin, and gets stored as fat or in muscles to be used as energy.

2. Relax more, exercise less. This conserves energy, or does it? You're not using up energy, but that's because this 'energy', i.e. fat, is lying dormant on your thighs/bingo wings/love handles, where it's not helping you.

3. Stimulate your body to burn existing fat. This uses up stored fat as energy by removing it from the aforementioned thighs/bingo wings/love handles; the reduction in excess layers of fat reveals the muscles beneath, resulting in a more toned, sculpted appearance. Reducing fat as well as exercising to build and tone muscles is important if your goals are aesthetic (you want to look toned) because otherwise your genuinely strong and toned stomach will be hidden from view by excess stored fat.

Guess which method we like to use at The Fit Mum Formula?

How we help you burn fat for energy

NUTRITION

A slice of cake, a bowl of cereal and milk, and a chicken and vegetable stir fry might all have the same calories, but do they all have the same effect on your body? No, they do not. Certain foods trigger hormonal and chemical responses that tell your body to store fat rather than burn it.

At The Fit Mum Formula I help you understand what to eat to encourage fat burning rather than storing, by supporting muscle tone and metabolism efficiency. By following the advice given you will experience increased energy, balanced blood sugar levels, improved focus and motivation and, of course, changes in body size, shape and tone, to give you a body you didn't think was possible without hours of dedication and effort.

EXERCISE

Think about Olympic sprinters, with their slim but perfectly shaped bodies, their strong, toned limbs, clear muscular definition, and glowing skin and eyes. Now think of many marathon runners – skinny and gaunt looking, with flabby skin hanging off their bones, prematurely aged skin, rubbery knees and tiny sagging bottoms. Why is this? (Hint: Google 'sprinter vs marathon runner') Think about how they exercise. A sprinter goes hell for leather for a few seconds, exerting every last drop of effort and energy, then they rest. A marathon runner will go for hours, steadily pacing themselves. It is exactly this reason that the two have such different body shapes, and at The Fit Mum Formula we know which we prefer.

Make this your new mantra:
Strong Is The New Skinny.

YOU DETERMINE YOUR OWN INTERVALS

The problem with traditional interval training, with set rest points and durations, is that they're much too hard for some people, yet not challenging enough for others. The solution? You take a rest when YOU need to, for as long as YOU need to, and join in again as soon as YOU are ready. Humans, like all animals, have this ability to self-regulate exercise, knowing when to push hard and when to rest by gauging how we feel. Work hard—rest hard—work hard, has been shown to be much more effective than pacing yourself continuously at a lower intensity, not only for burning fat but also for heart and lung efficiency, regulating hormones and minimising exercise induced stress. In short, it's great!

LIFESTYLE

Maybe you never realised how much your lifestyle has had as an effect on your body; you'd be forgiven for thinking it was all about food and exercise. But notice how you feel after a late night and you'll probably find you are hungrier the next day and are craving sugary, starchy foods. What about if it's a cloudy day? Or you spend hours in front of artificial light, such as the TV or computer, when the night sky outside is saying you should be asleep? Bad day? Stressed? Chocolate will cheer you up.

Well, there's a reason you react to all these scenarios with food: hormones. Not only that, but when you are stressed or sleep deprived your body will store more of the food you eat as fat, rather than using it to repair muscle or provide energy. It takes a lot of willpower to override these feelings, so I will teach you how to create the ideal environment and lifestyle that will not only make sticking to the programme so much easier, but it will also help your body to do much of the work for you!

THE FORMULA FUNDAMENTAL FIVE

1. Watch what you eat

Base meals and snacks on lean protein with plenty of low starch vegetables, salad, and some fruit, with limited amounts of starchy carbohydrates (no more than 1/5th of your plate at first). Eat dairy foods if they do not cause problems for you, such as digestive troubles. At least 30% of your calories should be made up of fat; don't ever cut fat out of your diet as this is not what causes health and weight issues. Avoid trans fats completely. Include plenty of unsaturated fats from oily fish, nuts, olives, avocado, etc. Don't be scared of saturated fats – recent research shows they're not nearly as evil as we once thought.

When reading food labels look beyond the calories; subtract the fibre from the total carbohydrates (per portion) to get net carbs, which tell you more about the effect it will have on blood sugar, since the more fibre there is the slower it will be released into your bloodstream and the lower the resulting insulin release. Now subtract the protein for the same portion size from the net carbs, as protein also slows food absorption, and the final number should be as low as possible, ideally less than 15, and negative numbers will impact blood sugar levels the least.

2. Watch when you eat

Eat 6 times a day; 3 meals plus 3 snacks. Never miss breakfast and eat within an hour of waking. Eat your evening meal a good 3 hours before bed, but have a little (protein based) snack before bed to prevent you waking from hunger and to help build muscle (and burn fat), as well as repair your body while you sleep. Try not to eat a big meal for 10 hours overnight; a 7pm meal then a 9pm or 10pm snack is a good routine. Note that as your body switches to burning fat as fuel you will find you can go longer between meals, eliminate snacks and go for longer without eating; you'll know when you're ready, you won't feel hungry or irritable if you haven't eaten in a while.

3. Know what works for you

You and your metabolic make up are individual; the number of calories you need, the percentage of carbohydrates and the way your body reacts to certain foods are different for each person. Work out whether you need to increase or decrease your starch intake from how you feel and whether you are toning up and losing fat. You want just enough to keep you satisfied and from having food cravings and energy dips, but not enough to hinder progress.

Avoid foods that are catalysts for your hunger and cravings and that result in dips in energy. Which foods do this and their effect on blood sugar levels are variable from person to person, but common culprits include coffee, energy drinks, sugar and artificial sweeteners, alcohol, gluten, dairy, nuts and nut butters, sweet snacks including dried fruit, and even low carb, healthy versions of cakes and treats.

On the other hand, small amounts of foods that satisfy a craving can reduce the risk of binging later, for example a couple of squares of dark chocolate instead of a whole chocolate bar when the urge gets too strong. Other foods which can satisfy cravings quickly for some people could be nuts or seeds (or nut/seed butters), high fat foods (e.g. avocado or creamy dips), sugar-free products such as sweets or chocolate, cheese, salty foods (e.g. parmesan cheese or olives), or sparkling flavoured water which is virtually calorie free if you buy sugar-free ones (it's the artificial sweeteners that can trigger cravings in some people). You can obviously only get away with a certain amount of these deterrent foods before they impact calorie intake, but in the short-term they can help stave off a binge, and over time, as your metabolism improves, cravings should lessen. You can see that there are overlaps and a food that is a catalyst for hunger and cravings for one person can be a deterrent against them for others. Get to know your body and how it reacts to certain foods.

4. Be selective with exercise and mindful of lifestyle

We Mums don't have time for hours in the gym or to go running for miles every day. And why would you want to when research shows it's not nearly as effective for fat loss as short bursts of intense exercise. Even one minute a day will show results over time. One minute! Doing the 30-minute high intensity workouts in The Fit Mum Formula's BodyBack programme the recommended 3–5 times a week should yield definitive results and changes in your strength, body shape and composition.

Walk as much as you can – to the shops, to school or nursery … – just 10 minutes round the block is better than nothing. And it doesn't matter what time of day you do it, the best time is the time that suits you.

Sleep as much as possible, and stress as little as possible; both make an impression on your metabolism and your body's ability to burn fat and build muscle. They also affect how you feel and ultimately how well you eat. High hunger, lots of cravings and low energy levels are your enemies and will eventually override willpower; avoid them with a vengeance.

5. Be perfect, but not all of the time

Organic, wholefoods from local producers are wonderful but not essential; you can get the same weight loss/fat burning/muscle building/metabolism supporting effects from foods at your local supermarket.

Exercising every day would be fantastic, but for many people it's not realistic. If your time to work out is 10pm on a Friday and Saturday night because the kids are in bed and you don't have to jump out of bed to get yourself and everyone ready for work/school the next day, then that's fine. The best time is the time that works for you, because then you'll stick to it.

Eat well, but don't beat yourself up over the odd cheat. Just like one 'good' meal won't make you slim, one 'bad' meal won't make you fat.

Have faith in yourself; be strong; be good; be perfect if you can, just not all of the time. Strive to make positive progress that improves both your health and your life. And if you have a slip up, just pick up where you left off and carry on, nothing is irreversible.

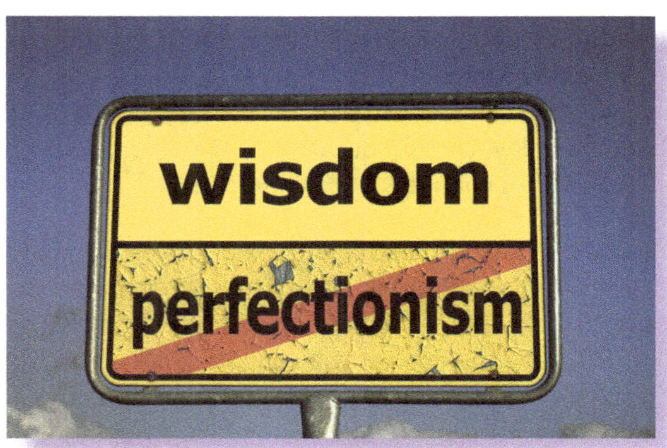

GOAL SETTING

The tradition of making resolutions at the turn of the New Year can be dated back 4,000 years to when ancient Babylonians would pray to their Gods in the hope of receiving strength, protection and good fortune over the coming twelve months. The Romans made similar promises to their God Janus, and medieval knights would reaffirm their chivalrous commitment to protecting their country each year. Given the seriousness that people put on their religious beliefs and the literal consequences that they believed might happen (terminal illness, death of family, failure of crops and starvation, or refused entry to Heaven, etc.), is it any wonder they stuck to their resolutions?

What resolutions come to mind among your friends and family? And what are the consequences if they are not stuck to?

I'm hazarding a guess you're probably not worried about going to Hell if you don't attend Zumba twice a week for the next six months.

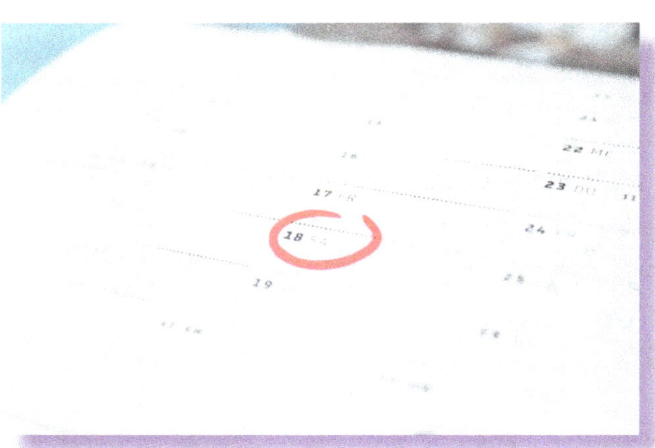

The most popular resolutions according to a 2011 Marist University poll were 'losing weight' at No. 1, followed by 'exercising more', 'being more careful with money', and 'quitting smoking'. Unfortunately, the psychologist Richard Wiseman of Bristol University found in a 2007 study that while 52% of people making New Year's Resolutions are confident they can stick it out, only 12% actually do.

Why?

Strategy. Or lack of. How is it possible, that after years of overeating/smoking/overspending, you reckon you can just wake up on January 1st (or next Monday) and suddenly have the means and willpower to change?

Sorry, but the human psyche doesn't work like that. It likes routine, habit, comfort; it is human nature to always 'take the path of least resistance' and give in (and have the fag/eat the chocolate bar/etc.). A resolution is placed on the 'to do' list without any idea of how it is going to be done. You wouldn't decide to move house without researching the best area to move to, getting a mortgage assessment, and finalising a sales contract first would you? You can't; without that planning you fail.

YOUR GOAL PLANNER

Read and action these before you begin

DECIDE ON YOUR GOALS

Trying to lose two stone in a month is neither healthy nor achievable. The more time you give yourself to lose the weight the better, but if you've left it too late (that holiday can't be changed!), still aim to lose around 0.5 kg a week (you might be able to stretch this to 1 kg a week if you have a lot of weight to lose). You might not be quite at your final weight goal by Goal Day, but at least you'll still have energy, and you'll have glossy hair and glowing skin. Dark rings under your eyes and a low mood (as well as irritability and low libido) are not worth starving yourself for.

SET A DATE

You want to lose a stone/run a 5k charity run/ etc. for when? For what? Maybe you're going on a warm holiday and want to feel confident in swimwear on the beach. Perhaps it's your birthday coming up and you want to mark it as the next stage in your life, to spend healthier, slimmer, fitter and happier. How long will you give yourself to reach your goal? Be realistic; the bigger the changes required, the longer they are likely take.

HAVE PROCESS GOALS AS WELL AS OUTCOME GOALS

The outcome is the end result: your goal weight; successfully completing a charity run; to stop feeling bloated all the time.

The process is the actions you do to get there. So for example, your goal might be: to eat 2 large handfuls of vegetables with every meal; to walk for 20 minutes every lunch break; to eat protein at every meal; or to do 10 minutes of lunges and press ups in front of the TV every night. Focussing on the actions needed to get to your goal make them easier to do simply because they're at the forefront of your mind. This is as opposed to the end goal, which might feel a little far away and out of reach when your first start your journey. Just hit your goals, for today, for this week, and the end results will come of their own accord, in time.

MAKE A MOOD BOARD

Studies show that making a visual dream or mood board taps into our subconscious and motivates us on a daily basis to do the things that take us further toward our goal. So if you're going somewhere hot for your holiday, buy a new bikini in the size you think you'll be after you've lost weight and hang it in your bedroom, where it reminds you why you're doing this. Make a picture board of things you need in your life to help you achieve your weight loss goals – a department store catalogue will have loads of inspirational ideas – pictures of trainers and workout clothes, weights, skipping ropes and other exercise equipment.

Or you can do it the 21st-century way and use Pinterest, which is essentially a digital mood board. Make a board for exercise, one for healthy food, one for motivational quotes and, importantly, one for other interests you have, because your diet and exercise should in no way be the only things you're focussing on.

ENROL HELP AND DELEGATE

You might ask your Mum to babysit and your neighbour to feed the cat when you're away, so why not ask people to help keep you on track with your diet and exercise plans too? Perhaps a friend would also like to lose weight or get fit and could work out with you. Ask if anyone has any healthy recipes they can share with you, and ask your Mum nicely to please stop bringing the biscuits out every time you visit her! Studies show that people with good peer support are more successful in sticking to plans and achieving goals, both short and long term.

SLEEP!

It might surprise you to learn that diet and exercise aren't the only things that matter. Sleep is when your body builds muscle (you won't 'bulk up' but it does make you look toned, which is what most women think looks nice), burns fat and recovers from exercise. Not enough sleep means you'll be hungrier and have less energy and willpower the next day, so you're more likely to skip workouts and eat comfort food. Stress and lack of sleep also deplete willpower and the stress hormone cortisol encourages fat storage around your middle. Yoga and massage are great stress relievers, as is walking (especially in 'green' areas), which of course doubles up as gentle exercise.

PLAN FOR FAILURE

This isn't being negative, it's being prepared. What do you do when you have no energy on a Friday night and really want a takeaway? Have you picked out some less calorific options that won't completely derail you? Chinese chop suey (protein with beansprouts) and Indian dry chicken tandoori (as opposed to in a sauce), with a bag of salad from the corner shop, are two of my favourite choices when I want to still eat well.

How about at your kids' birthday parties? Can you eat a healthy meal before so you don't end up picking at loads of sandwiches, crisps and cake all afternoon? Anticipate tricky situations arising (because they will) and know in advance how to deal with them.

BE ACCOUNTABLE

If you're relying only on yourself to make yourself do x/y/z, you're on wobbly ground. While ultimately you have to find the strength and motivation to do this by yourself, for yourself, it's probably a good idea to have someone keeping you on track, at least at first. Maybe you and a friend can text each other each time you've done a workout. Or if you use social media then post what you're up to; you'll probably find people chip in with praise and motivation. The same goes for when you're struggling; tell someone that box of chocolates in the cupboard is driving you mad, and someone will remind you why you should have just one rather than all of them.

PLAN REWARDS

Not just about reaching your goal (which in itself is rewarding), what non-food rewards will you give yourself? We do sticker charts for children because they really do work! It doesn't have to be extravagant or expensive. Maybe you've not had a haircut in a while, or if your clothes no longer fit then you'll need to get a few basics in your new size.

Your goal setting checklist

- Make a resolution because it's something that is really important to you, not just something you vaguely feel you should do. If your heart isn't in it, you won't succeed.

- Don't change too many things at once. Long-term habits take concentration if you are to succeed in breaking them, so focus on one goal at a time.

- Go For Goal. Success is much more likely if very specific goals are set: losing 'a pound a week' or 'being able to run for 10 minutes without stopping', rather than simply to 'lose weight' or 'run more'.

- Strength in numbers. Make your goals public and seek support from those around you, whether that be encouragement from friends and family, or joining a support network. Some online coaching programmes – including my own BodyBack programme – encourage social support through online forums and chat areas.

- Write a 'Business Plan' with weekly and monthly goals, potential areas for difficulties and failures, and preventative measures against these.

- Have what you need, like workout training shoes? Sports bra? Clean, appropriate clothing? Don't let details like this become an excuse, have them ready!

- Monitor progress and measure where you're at against your 'business plan' once a week at least.

- Reward success. If you made a significant achievement at work you'd be pretty annoyed if you didn't receive the deserved recognition for your hard work. Though, choose a reward that supports your goals instead of opposes them – a massage instead of a takeaway pizza, in other words.

- Expect the Unexpected – and deal with it. You might be presented with a cake on your birthday. Have a slice. Don't eat another four once everyone has gone home.

- Expect to fail – sometimes. Being 100% perfect all the time is unrealistic; you will fail if you hope to always be perfect. Be 100% perfect 80% of the time.

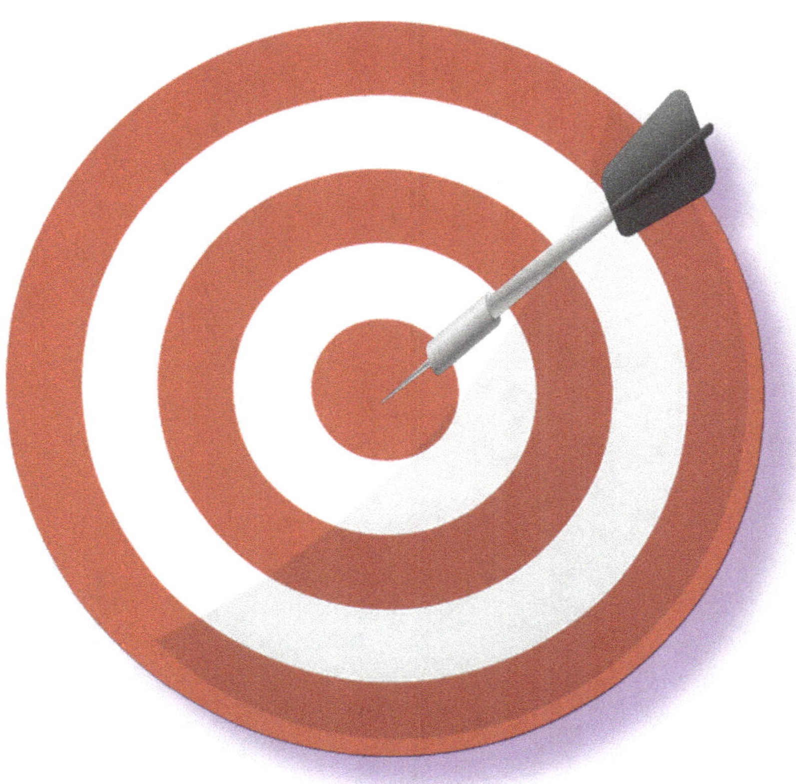

TRAINING

WHY YOU PREFER TO SIT

The reasons you don't get enough of the right types of exercise are 50% knowledge ('what should I do?'), 50% practical ('how do I find time to do it?') and 100% mindset – that last one because with the right mindset you can make pretty much anything happen and work for you, for the most part. We'll be covering more on mindset later.

Call me stubborn, overambitious, idealistic, if you like. But my motto in life has always been that it's not about IF you can do something, only a matter of HOW. But before you tell me 'But I really can't get to the gym – I get home at 8pm and have to put my kids to bed', etc. etc., I'm not talking about trying to do things you can't do.

I'm talking about finding a way around this problem, finding a solution to the barriers, so that you can still achieve the same results.

Let's look at some of the most common reasons people don't exercise, or don't exercise enough.

You dislike exercise

I know this already. If you loved exercise enough to have it high on your priority list you would find a way to fit it in, believe me you would. It's OK if you don't like exercise. You probably have negative memories, and emotions attached to those memories.

Did I ever tell you about my experiences at boarding school? I've always thrived in creative, agility sports – gymnastics, trampolining, ice skating, dancing. But running? Let's just say I figured out that if I just made it round the field during cross country I could sit in the woods for 20 minutes before running back, for a realistically timed finish. Turns out I had undiagnosed asthma all my life, which no doubt didn't help, which is triggered by damp air – dewy Cotswold fields and woodland come to mind. To this day running (by which I mean jogging; sprinting I love, sometimes) is a mental barrier for me, even though I have an inhaler on standby and the knowledge that I am, in fact, very fit. The answer? I don't run. I do other stuff.

On the other hand some people will never like any sort of exercise. It's rare, but it happens. In this situation you have to evaluate what you really want. Sometimes we have to do things we don't want to do to get the things we do want, or to avoid the things we don't want. You go to work because you want to treat you family to a holiday. You brush your teeth because you don't want bad breath and rotten teeth. You do it for the end result, not just the process.

Not enough time

Everybody has 24 hours in a day. You are spending those hours working, doing household chores, caring for children, shopping, eating, and hopefully sleeping! You might watch a bit of TV. All these things (except maybe the TV) have to be done. But if you leave exercise at the bottom of the priority list, well, when was the last time you got to the bottom of your to-do list?! I remember clearly the last time I did; before Aurora was born, 8 years ago! If you choose to exercise (note I didn't say want to, that's a separate matter), it has to be in your diary like a business meeting, and prioritised, prepared for, and attended on time.

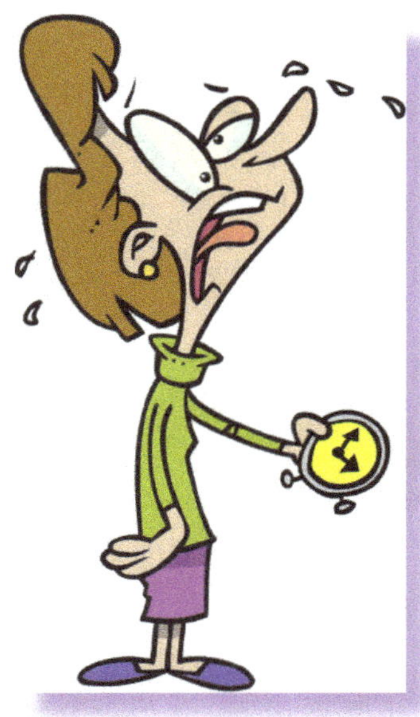

You can't get to the gym

Hardly anyone actually keeps going to the gym. Why the poor attendance rates? Most people start with lofty goals, with the best of intentions to go to classes four nights a week and again on weekend mornings. But very few people have the time to commit to this, and so, believing they need to do huge amounts of exercise to get fitness results, view a more modest approach as pointless, and ultimately give up entirely.

I was never a gym goer (in fact I wasn't really an exerciser once I stopped dancing, apart from walking loads and having a job on my feet as a beauty therapist). But once I had my first baby I realised that doing anything for myself, child free, let alone the gym, was going to be a challenge. I didn't have a weight problem but I wasn't very fit and certainly wasn't strong (a classic 'skinny fat'). It's exactly the reason The Fit Mum Formula came about, a mum-life friendly way to connect with other Mums with the same goals, learn new skills, and get more energy and the body you want, even if your life doesn't revolve around the gym and going to classes.

You don't own any equipment

Gym machines, like treadmills and leg presses, are very expensive (usually in the thousands of pounds) and take up a lot of space. Even a barbell and a few weights are awkward to store. If you want to inject some variety and increase the intensity then a pair of dumb-bells are a good place to start, or a kettlebell if you know what to do with it. But honestly? You don't need equipment if your goal is to lose weight and tone up. Your body is the weight – and I'm not being sarcastic here – even a very slim person is heavy enough to provide resistance when used in the right way.

I'm now going to address each of these barriers in more detail and show you how you can overcome them.

BEING MORE ACTIVE DOESN'T HAVE TO MEAN FORMAL EXERCISE

What if you could get more activity into your life without forking out for a gym membership in the first place? After all, many people already put themselves in debt from overspending on Christmas presents and festivities, so adding to this with an expensive (and unused) gym membership on January 2nd seems like a poor manoeuvre to me.

10 ways to be more active at home today for free

Here's 10 simple ways you can get more exercise into your life without spending a penny. Will they make you an Olympian? Probably not. But do them all as much as possible and they add up surprisingly fast. Every little really does help.

1. MAKE A STANDING DESK

Notice I didn't say 'buy' a standing desk. Because that costs money, takes time, and you might not have space for it at home or be allowed one at work. Simply place your computer or laptop on a raised surface, such as a dressing table or sideboard, and work, shop online or reply to emails while standing up. You'll burn more calories and your back will definitely thank you. Sitting all day means we're not using our posterior chain muscles – the back, buttocks, and hamstrings – so they get weak, which can lead to backache and hip problems. Standing engages these muscles with hardly any effort on your part.

2. TAKE EVERY OPPORTUNITY TO USE THE STAIRS

We know this one and when the choice is between escalator, lift or stairs we know which we should be doing. But what about at home? In my house we have downstairs loo, but I never use it – going to the upstairs bathroom is one more flight of stairs to climb that I take advantage of! And if you're faced with escalators only (such as on the London Underground), don't stand on the right – walk quickly up the left hand side and give your legs a fantastic workout – that's a lot of stairs!

3. CARRY SHOPPING BAGS BY HAND

Heavy handbags and rucksacks slung over the shoulder are not at all good for postural muscles; they encourage a rounded back and shoulders and create an imbalance between the two sides of your body. In fact, you can see people who always carry heavy bags on the same shoulder when you do a postural analysis – they're lopsided!

On the other hand, carrying shopping bags in from the car uses all the muscles in your body to stabilise you. Hold the bags by the handles with your arms hanging down by your sides, with roughly equal weight in each hand, and carrying as many bags as possible. There's actually an exercise called Farmer's Walks that is exactly this, but usually using weights in a gym.

4. GET A PEDOMETER

OK, I know I said 'for free', but you can get pedometers for under £1, including postage, on eBay so I think that counts! We all know we should be walking more, but do you really know how many steps you take each day? Fitness trackers and pedometers have this brilliant (psychological) way of making you more aware of trying to walk as much as possible. The numbers don't lie and you'll find yourself pacing the corridors while on the phone to make sure you hit that 10,000 steps daily target.

5. CLEAN YOUR HOUSE

This job isn't nearly so tedious if you know it's saving you a gym membership and getting your body moving. Put some effort in and give it some welly; you'll get the job done quicker and the physical benefits will be greater. Stretch up to clean the tops of indoor windows, squat and crouch to wipe the skirting boards or scrub the floor, tone up your shoulder muscles with a good resistance workout wiping and polishing, and hoover and mop at speed to get your heart rate up!

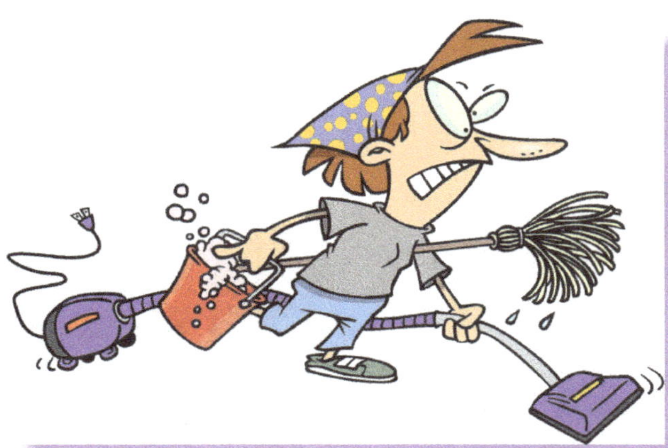

6. SET A TIMER

Set an alarm to go off every 15 minutes, and when it beeps get up and do something active. If you're at work it could be as simple as delivering paperwork to someone's desk, doing some photocopying, making tea for yourself and a colleague, or taking a phone call while pacing outside. At home or in more private areas you can really go for it. I've been known to do 10 burpees every 15 minutes throughout the day when it had been raining all week and I had been doing the school run in the car. I was really feeling the exhilaration of exercise by the end of the day, and I definitely was more productive working at home from all the 'mini breaks'.

7. HAVE A CLEAR OUT

We tend to use the phrase spring cleaning, but I prefer to have a good sort through all our 'stuff' right after Christmas, as old, broken, unwanted junk gets replaced with shiny new presents. This is especially good if you have kids who a) own a tonne of plastic rubbish they never play with, and b) grow out of their clothes fast. You'll be amazed how all that sorting, bagging, lifting, emptying and tidying involves almost every body movement – bending, stretching, lifting, dragging and carrying. It's immensely satisfying to suddenly have space in your cupboards once more, and if you give unbroken things to charity you'll be doing a good turn too.

8. WATCH TV

Really?! What I mean is, do something while you're watching TV. Alternate bodyweight squats with push ups and with sit ups, lie in a plank position, or do some yoga or pilates movements and stretches. It'll relax you at the same time as tiring your muscles, so you might find you sleep better too.

9. WEED THE GARDEN

I would say 'do some gardening', but since I have trouble keeping a houseplant alive I'd be a bit of a hypocrite. But weeding, gathering up leaves, trimming hedges and all those 'don't need to know about plants' jobs I can do, and so can you.

10. TAKE AN INVIGORATING SHOWER

There's a time and a place for a long hot bath, in fact I try to do this if I've done a tough workout that day, and I add Epsom salts or Magnesium flakes to the water to help relax my muscles. But the rest of the time stand up, do some body brushing, use a body scrub, and keep moving all the while. You save water too. A tip for a good night's sleep is to finish with 30 seconds of cold water. It sounds horrendous but the trick is to have the water hot enough most of the time that the cold water is almost a relief. Trust me you'll have the best sleep of your life.

So there you have it, no excuses needed about lack of time, money for the gym or not owning any equipment, it turns out all the things you need to get more active are already right in your own home!

EXERCISE DOESN'T HAVE TO TAKE A LOT OF TIME

Work, studies, children, parents, significant others, family life … it's no wonder we don't have all the time we'd like to dedicate to exercise. It's seems pretty reasonable to put your lack of fitness, or being a little larger than you'd like, down to not being able to work out enough to get results.

Or perhaps you are pounding the pavements every day – jogging before work, group class after work, long cycle rides every weekend – yet no matter how many miles or minutes you add up you still can't seem to make progress!

Work smarter not harder

I'm going to let you in on a little secret that will change your approach to exercise, and save you a load of time and effort while we're at it.

You need to stop doing *more,* and start doing it *better.*

You need to work out *smarter*, not *harder.*

You see, when it comes to getting results, quality or exercise can matter as much, and often more, than quantity.

THE PROBLEM WITH MORE EXERCISE

For one, this takes more time. Time most of us don't have, and that is a big enough problem to discount any other factors, since if you can't do the exercise needed, you definitely won't get results.

Secondly, our bodies can only cope with so much stress and, believe it or not, exercise is definitely stressful on your body. Cortisol is released, and the longer you work out, the more cortisol there is to wreak havoc on your body, since it is linked to everything from mental health problems to adrenal fatigue, diabetes, heart disease and more.

Hunger also increases with more exercise, so if 50 lengths of the pool leads to consuming a latte and a piece of carrot cake the size of your head in the café afterwards, you'll most likely be undoing any calorie burning you've just achieved.

THE SMARTER WAY TO EXERCISE

High Intensity Interval Training (HIIT) is fast becoming the go-to method for people wanting maximum results in minimum time. The, so-called, intervals consist of a few seconds (up to 90 but can be as little as 10 seconds) of difficult exercises, where you put maximum all-out effort in, followed by a few seconds, or even minutes, of rest or very low intensity work, before launching into the next 'intense' work round, and so the cycle repeats for your chosen duration to complete the workout.

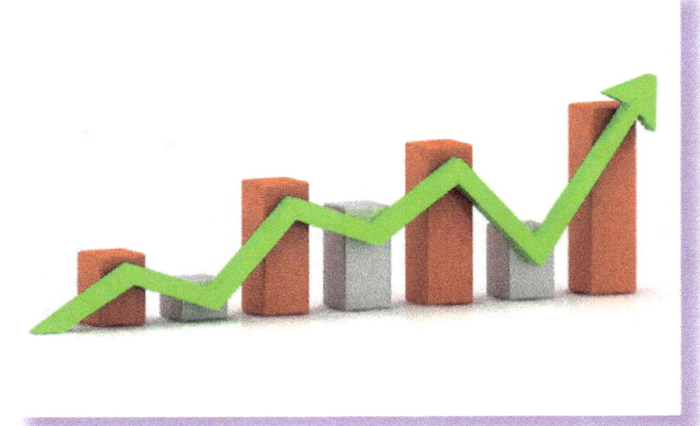

The sheer effort you'll be putting into your bouts of exercise during each work interval means that workouts will only be, on average, around 20 minutes long, sometimes as short as 10 minutes. If you're managing to keep going like this for longer than 45 minutes then, quite frankly, you're not putting enough effort into it.

And that's the other beauty of this method. The fitter and stronger you get, the more effort you put in, the more reps you can do in your work time, or the more weight you can use if you choose to. You can make regressions or progressions to exercises depending on your level, and adjust the work and rest times to suit you. For example, someone very new to fitness might do 30 seconds of box push ups followed by 60 seconds rest, then repeat. A more advanced exerciser could do 60 seconds of decline push ups followed by 30 seconds rest.

THE BENEFITS OF HIIT

HIIT training has been shown to improve aerobic and anaerobic fitness, blood pressure, cardiovascular health, insulin sensitivity (which helps the exercising muscles use glucose more readily for fuel to make energy), cholesterol profiles, abdominal fat and body weight while maintaining muscle mass. It can be used for all sport and fitness goals, can be progressed or regressed to suit the person doing it, and it really does yield impressive results in very little time.

Aerobic and cardiovascular health

In 2011 Dr Niels Vollard at Bath University conducted a trial in which subjects did short (10–20 second) bursts of intense cycling, sandwiched between a couple of minutes gentle cycling to warm up and cool down. Both male and female subjects showed marked improvements in aerobic fitness and insulin sensitivity.

Another study, conducted by McMaster University in Ontario, showed that overweight or obese individuals who performed just 60 seconds of all-out intermittent exercise per week for 6 weeks improved their endurance levels by about 12%, had better blood pressure levels, improved muscle activity, and the male participants also improved their blood sugar control.

Muscle building and fat burning

HIIT makes your muscles produce new and more efficient mitochondria, the tiny power factories in your cells that convert glucose into useable energy. The more mitochondria you have, the more power they produce and the more fat and sugar they consume.

The stress caused by HIIT also leads to the release of large amounts of catecholamines – which are hormones such as adrenaline and noradrenaline – that target fat cells, particularly those in the abdomen.

Calorie advantage

The type of exercise you do also appears to affect hunger levels and therefore the amount of calories consumed following working out.

An Australian study involving overweight men in their 20s and early 30s found that the men ate fewer calories after doing very high-intensity workouts (594 calories) than after moderate exercise. Fewer calories were also consumed the following day; 2,000 after HIIT, compared to 2,300 after a session of moderate intensity exercise.

Short and sweet

The deal is that if you're going to work out for such a short time, you've got to make it worth it, putting in maximum effort and as high intensity as you can manage. No pacing yourself, you shouldn't be able to hold a conversation and it should feel like the hardest workout you ever did. But knowing it's over after a mere one minute should make it feel that much more worthwhile and manageable. And you should probably aim to do it every other day, perhaps first thing in the morning to get it over with (though whenever suits you is fine). If you want to do it every day a trick is to use different muscles on each day so that you're giving each muscle group at least a day to recover.

SET INTERVALS OR SELF-PACED?

There are two ways to implement interval training.

The first is set, timed intervals that are predetermined, so you decide from the outset that you would exercise for 60 seconds followed by 60 seconds rest, or whatever you decide is appropriate. This is the way most people do interval training and, so long as the exercise choices, levels, and interval times are appropriate to your needs and fitness level, it can work well.

The issue is that it can be tricky to figure out the perfect system for you without a lot of trial and error.

I prefer a method called rest-based training, whereby the person working out is trusted to define their own rest intervals judging on how they feel while working out. In essence, you work as hard as you can with maximum effort and good technical form, but when you're feeling too tired to go all out, or your technique starts to get sloppy, you rest, then pick up where you left off when you feel capable of putting in maximum effort once more.

Is this a recipe for slacking off or pushing too hard? Not so. The RPE scale (rate of perceived exertion, essentially, how do you feel on a scale of 1-10?)

used by trainers to assess how hard a person feels they are working is a common example of how people are in touch with how they feel. Studies show RPE to be remarkably in line with heart rate when monitored simultaneously.

The result is that you get a workout that's not too easy (not enough stimulation to make progressions) and not too hard, which can lead to injury as well as stress-induced hormonal disruptions that come with their own storm of metabolic catastrophe. You get a workout that's the perfect level to suit you. In fact, studies show that defining your own intervals leads to as good as, if not better, outcomes than the traditional set method.

Not for everyone

For the very unfit, overweight, or people with medical conditions, working out at this intensity may not be possible at first. If you are extremely unfit it would be wise to have a medical check-up before starting any form of exercise.

However, intense is a relative term and if walking briskly for 20 seconds followed by standing still for 30 seconds and repeating that pattern a few times is intense, then that's a starting point and you can work toward more difficult exercises. Studies of nearly 5,000 patients with a history of heart conditions and strokes have found HIIT to be perfectly safe.

YOU DON'T NEED THE GYM

The best exercise is the one you enjoy and the one you stick to. Consistency, that is keeping to a realistic schedule and very rarely missing a workout, is more important than what you actually choose to do for that workout.

That being said, most women already have enough on their plate with work, studying, children, etc. So anything that can be done in as short a time as possible while still making progress makes sense. I prefer HIIT for this reason, and that is what I coach on my The Fit Mum Formula 'BodyBack' programme.

HIIT can be done anywhere, including indoors, with no equipment needed, so it's perfect for the winter months when it's cold and dark outside.

60-SECOND DAILY WORKOUTS

When you're really busy (and who's life isn't these days) exercise might be the last of your priorities. If you can't commit to going to the gym three times a week, or going for a half hour run every day, then you're not going to benefit, so why bother?

Well, it turns out that short bursts of exercise have more impact than you think on your health, fitness, weight and body composition.

Of course, these great results HIIT gets aren't to prove you needn't bother working out more than 60 seconds, or that for the best body composition or performance goals you don't need to obviously put in more work than that. But if 60 seconds is literally all you can spare, do it the right way and you'll get a surprising amount from one minute a day.

Try these 60 second workouts for a whole body routine spread out over the week.

All the workouts can be done at home or outside, with no or minimal equipment, since I doubt you'll be wanting to go to the gym for 60 seconds a day!

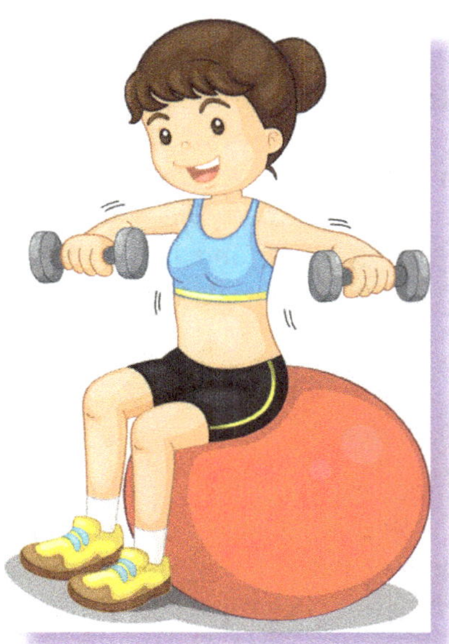

DAY 1 — PRESS UPS

20 seconds of full body press ups, 10 seconds rest, 20 seconds full body press ups, 10 seconds mountain climbers.

Make it harder: make them plyometric press ups.

DAY 2 — SPRINT INTERVALS

10 seconds sprint, 10 seconds rest, repeat 6 times.

Make it harder: increase to 20 seconds sprint, 10 seconds rest, and do it twice.

DAY 3 — DUMB-BELL SQUAT AND PRESS

Do a full minute, squatting as low as you can.

Make it harder: use heavier weights.

DAY 4 — BURPEES

15 seconds of burpees, as fast as you can with proper form, 5 seconds rest, repeat three times.

Make it harder: hold a dumb-bell in each hand while you do them.

DAY 5 — JUMP SQUATS

Try to do a whole minute of jump squats. Take a 5 second rest after 30 seconds if you need to.

Make it harder: hold a dumb-bell in each hand while you jump.

DAY 6 — BICYCLES

Go as fast as you can for a full minute while getting your knees as close to your elbows as possible (no half bicycles!).

Make it harder: wrist and ankle weights mean your core needs to work even harder.

DAY 7 — THREE-WAY SHOULDER BLAST

10 seconds bent over dumb-bell rows, 10 seconds tricep extensions, 10 seconds reverse dumb-bell flys. Repeat all.

Make it harder: increase the weight of the dumb-bell.

PLAYGROUND WORKOUT

If you've got small kids like I do, you'll know how hard it is to find 'me time' for simple things like a bath by yourself, let alone making time for exercise. Even if your kids are at school during the day most people work or have other commitments that get in the way of exercise. But here's an idea you might not have considered:

Do your workout with the kids, in the playground!

Why are playgrounds so great?

As a Mum to 3-year-old and 6-year-old girls I'm no stranger to parks and playgrounds. Even with a new climbing frame in our garden the girls still love to play on new equipment, and bumping into other kids to play with there, too. The fresh air does wonders for 'blowing the cobwebs away', as my mother says, by which she means destressing, expending pent up angst and/or energy, which is good for the immune system. And sunlight helps our bodies produce those all-important Vitamin D stores that we tend to lack in the northern hemisphere.

I admit I'm more of a 'do-er' than a 'sitter' and resent having to keep still for too long, but even appreciating that other parents might appreciate some rest, I regularly witness parents (mostly women, but the theory applies to men too) sitting on benches for an entire hour moaning about their thighs/bingo wings/etc., discussing what boot camp/class/trendy diet they plan to start next week.

If only these ladies would look up and see what their little ones are accomplishing on the free equipment in this free playground that is open all hours, they'd see that a workout could be easier to fit in than they think!

GET TRIM ON A TRIM TRAIL

Some parks actually have trim trails, which are essentially playground-like structures designed for physical activity (aka exercise) for both adults and kids alike; your local council should be able to tell you where your local ones are. Monkey bars, rope bridges and nets to climb will all challenge your body in ways you wouldn't do in everyday life, even with 'conventional' exercise. OK so children have youth, great flexibility, a lack of injury history and typically bags of energy on their side, but much of their vitality can indeed be attributed to the fact that they get out there and use their body, simply by playing.

But even if your park only has a few basic pieces of equipment, knowing how you can use them can provide a workout to rival any expensive gym equipment, and your kids will love that you're getting involved and playing with them!

HERE ARE SOME IDEAS YOU CAN TRY IN YOUR LOCAL PLAYGROUND.

Steps incline/decline push-ups

For an easier push-up, keep your feet on the ground and place your hands at the outer edges of a step so that your body is at an angle. Lower your chest toward the steps then raise, repeat for however many reps you can manage with the full range of motion. For a harder version, place your feet on a step with your hands on the ground so now your head is pointing toward the ground, then do the push-ups from this position.

Monkey bars

This one should be self-explanatory. Like with pull-ups and chin-ups (but with the help of momentum gained while keeping moving), these challenge the arm and back muscles. Plus, it's extremely satisfying getting to the other side without having to drop down half way across!

Fireman's pole

Up not down! Make sure the pole and your hands are dry and free of grease (a small towel makes a useful playground accessory, especially if it's been raining), and grip the pole with your hands. Use your hands, feet, knees and arms as necessary to climb up the pole as high as you can go, then climb back down the same way, trying not to 'cheat' by sliding down instead!

Bench tricep dips

Find an unoccupied bench and, facing away from the bench, place your hands on the seat and either bend your knees at right angles or straighten them out in front (your choice), keeping your bottom raised off the ground. Use your tricep muscles to lower your bottom toward the ground then raise it back up again. Repeat for 10–15 reps.

Swing split squat

Stand with your back to the swing and lift one foot up behind you to place on the swing. Place your hand on your hips and bend your front leg, keeping your foot flat on the ground and knee aligned over your foot, allowing your back knee to lower as you do. Return to the starting position and repeat for 10 reps before switching and doing the same on the other leg.

Pull-ups/chin-ups

The basic structure of most climbing frames is poles, or beams of metal or wood, which are perfect for doing pull-ups and chin-ups (watch for splinters on wooden frames). Find a horizontal pole that you can comfortably grip with both hands while standing on the ground. Squeeze your shoulder blades together and use your back and arm muscles to pull the bar toward you, raising your feet off the ground, then lower. If you can't manage a full rep, find a bar you can climb up to so that you begin at the top with your chin aligned with the bar, then practice lowering yourself in a controlled manner.

These are just some of the many ways you can use a playground to create a great workout, what other creative ideas can you come up with to keep things fun and interesting?

P.S. if you're not a parent or don't look after children often then don't let that stop you – there's no age limit on most playground equipment, so as long as you're not stopping other kids from playing there's no reason you can't be the 'big kid' and get climbing too! You might find during school/nursery hours are quieter, so the equipment you want to use is more likely to be free.

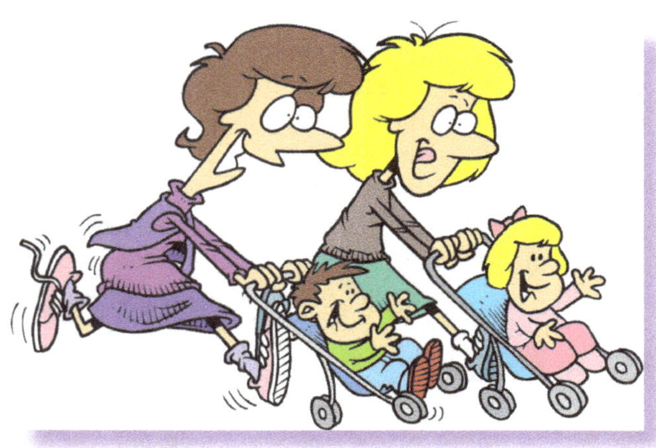

YOU DON'T NEED EQUIPMENT

Having a trusty list of bodyweight exercises in your repertoire is vital to enable you to get a good workout in, wherever you are and whatever circumstances you're in.

Getting to the gym isn't always possible. Holidays, family to look after, and work schedules mean that being able to work out at home is much more realistic for most people. Yet, not everyone wants to buy, or has room for, lots of exercise equipment to keep at home.

This is where a list of bodyweight exercises, which you can mix and match depending on what you want to do that day, can provide all you need in terms of getting in a full body workout that's both effective and convenient.

Don't be fooled into thinking bodyweight exercises are too easy. In fact one of their great benefits is how you can progress and regress exercises by changing reps, sets, position or lever length to make an exercise easier or harder depending on your strength and fitness levels.

It's best to get in a variety of exercises over the week for each body part, so that you get a full body workout and your muscles develop evenly with no imbalances or weak areas, which can lead to overcompensating with stronger muscles and is more likely to lead to overuse injuries.

There are literally hundreds of bodyweight exercise possibilities and many variations, progressions and regressions for each one.

The exercises provided in this book are all body weight exercises. If they're becoming too easy (because you're getting so fit and strong!), do a harder variation, do more reps in the same amount of time (go faster!), rest less often and for shorter durations, or consider investing in a low priced set of ankle and wrist strap weights, or a set of dumb-bells to hold, which in my experience are a great tool to have on hand that don't cost the earth or take up much space.

TRAINING ONLINE, FROM HOME

If you're one of the busy Mums who cite no time to exercise and/or childcare as your reasons for not getting in the workouts you know you should be doing, then online training is probably right for you.

Even if you are able to get to the gym, it might not be as good an option for you as training online at home.

Gyms, and even forking out for a personal trainer (PT), come with downsides. Most people aren't aware of the best way to spend their time when they are at the gym – what exercises will get them closer to their goals – meaning they go week after week but don't see results.

PTs overcome this by giving you a personalised plan (or at least they should be, not all PTs are created equal unfortunately), but are only with you for around 1–3 hours per week. What about the other 167 hours in a week? What then?

Online training has grown enormously in the past few years. In fact when The Fit Mum Formula first launched in 2013 we were one of the first, at least in the UK; a fact I'm rather proud of, ☺.

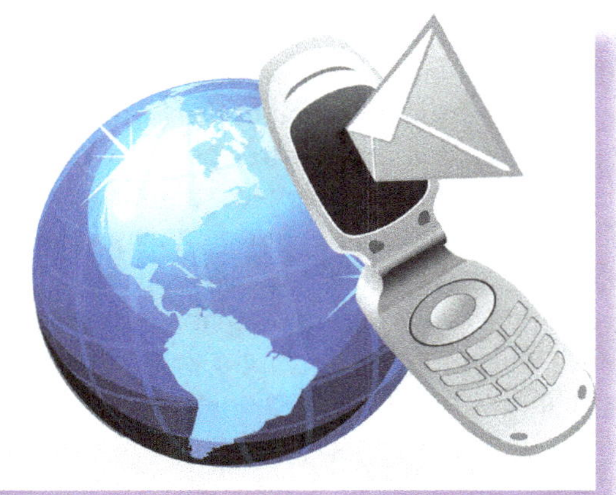

Internet, email, Facebook groups and forums, blogs, membership portals and dedicated workout plan software means that wherever you (or your coach) are, you can access help and information anytime you need it.

This means that you have the resources and support you need, to keep you on track 24/7, and as a result are much more likely to reach your goals, and in less time.

10 benefits to training online, from home

TIME SAVING

Travelling to the gym takes time. Parking the car, changing clothes, finding a locker … You can skip the lot if your workouts are done at home. I don't even bother 'getting changed' properly – if you follow me on social media you'll know my favourite workout outfit is my pyjama bottoms and a sports bra!

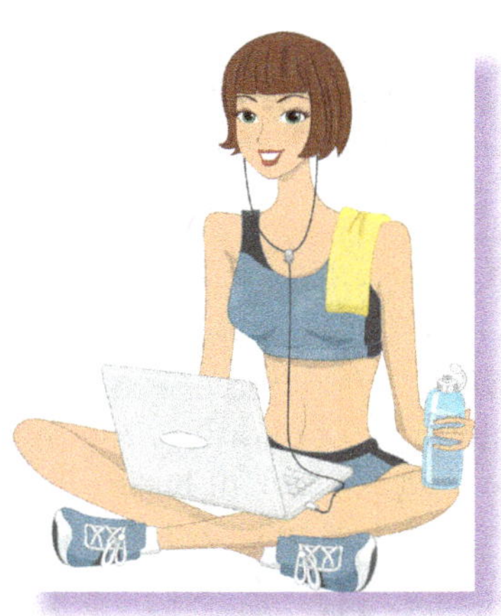

GOOD VALUE

With no special equipment or workout clothing you're already saving a few quid, but the real saving comes from the (rising) costs of gym memberships and PT services, especially if you're tied into a contract you don't end up using. Having the support of an online coach is often much more cost effective, since there are few overheads for the coach to pay (PT's pay rent to gyms), and the flexibility means more clients can be taken on than with in-person training. There are some very high priced 'transformation' coaches around, but I've yet to see one who can justify the thousands (literally) they command each month. Personally, I see this as an opportunity to pass those benefits on to you by being able to charge a much more reasonable monthly price, while still getting you to reach your goals.

NO ONE ELSE TO JUDGE

A strange concept people have is that they have to 'get fit' before they can go to the gym. Isn't this what exercising is supposed to do, not the other way round? But it really stems from insecurities, a fear of being judged by others further along the health/weight/fitness goal path than you. You should never be made to feel insecure stepping into any fitness facility, it's unacceptable. However, sometimes these insecurities come from within our own head, and while this needs to be challenged, training at home gets round this while still enabling you to make progress.

NO ONE TO HOG THE EQUIPMENT

Applicable more to those who work out with big heavy weights or machines (and why else would you use a gym?), imagine having a plan, workout template, your preferred workout to do, all prepped and ready, only to find that the local college are teaching their trainee PT's that day, there's a special offer on to use the gym, or half the machines are 'out of order'. Your home is your private gym, and equipment based workouts can easily be switched for effective and select body weight exercises in most cases, especially if your goal is simply to lose weight and tone up (which is most Mums' goal).

FLEXIBLE

No one plan suits everyone. No timescale is right for every person. You go on holiday, change jobs, have sick children, move house. Having a strict meal and workout plan won't work in these circumstances. Paid for three times a week training but need to take the dog to the vet that morning? You are unlikely get a refund. But with online training that's fine – just fit it in when it's a better time for you; when you get home from the appointment, in your hotel room, before the school run, heck, even at 2am if you want to (night shift workers?!).

ACCOUNTABILITY

You can't see an in-person trainer at all hours, every day. They have other clients to train, inflexible schedules to stick to, and places to be. While this is still partly true for online coaches – I still have work to do – the flexibility means I can stay in touch with clients whenever they need me, and technology makes keeping in touch with many people in less time possible. For you this means you don't get forgotten, and likewise, the regular contact keeps you on track and accountable, so you're less likely to deviate from what you need to be doing.

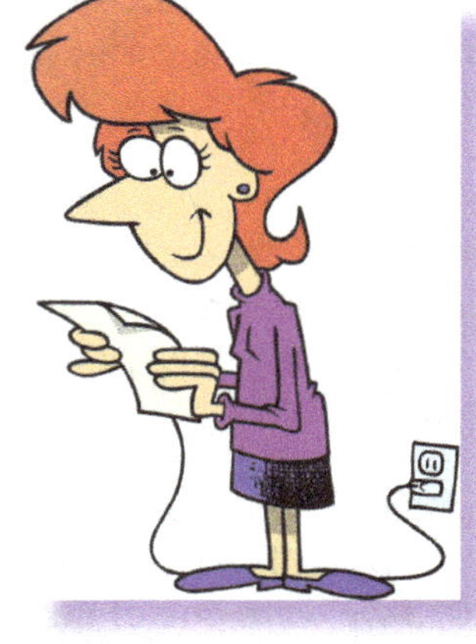

UPSKILLING

Let's get this straight; with any trainer, on or offline, you're not paying for information. We have information overload in the form of the internet. What you get with a good coach is relevant, informed, personalised information that is applicable to you. Understanding why your coach is telling you certain things makes you more likely to agree and follow through with instructions, which in turn will, you guessed it, get you closer to your goals, in less time. Never is delivery of information easier than online, where articles and links to specific information are just a click away and can be sent to you in seconds.

MONITORING PROGRESS

Like the benefits of flexibility and accountability, adjusting and tweaking your plan is important to make sure it a) is working, and b) works within your life and circumstances. This is much easier if you have resources and contact with your trainer to help you tweak as and when necessary, rather than having to wait until you next see them.

UNDERSTANDING

While a concern might be that a coach you've never met won't fully understand you, this couldn't be further from the truth. Not only do platforms like Facebook mean that people put much of their life online anyway, but the regular contact and community created between myself and all my clients mean we get to know each other far better than if we only saw each other a couple of times a week. I've formed fantastic bonds with many of my clients, and this understanding means I can better determine exactly what they need from me, at any given time.

SUPER EFFECTIVE

If you thought exercising at home wasn't as effective as going to the gym or a class, then you've clearly not yet seen or experienced the results that my clients, with the right type of training, are getting. In fact home workouts are the only thing I've ever done since having children (my eldest daughter Aurora is 7 at the time of writing). Following along to a DVD is an option, but it's a stab in the dark since it might not be right for you, and you obviously don't get the support, accountability and help with other things, like diet and meal planning, that you do with a coach.

For the busy Mum who wants to lose weight and tone up but either can't get to the gym, or isn't getting the results hoped for, online training is an option that's flexible enough to fit into your crazy Mum-life while still getting the body and body confidence you want.

To discuss whether online training is right for visit **www.thefitmumformula.com** to book your free diet and exercise planning call, and whether you're a good fit or not, I guarantee you'll come away from the call with some simple, actionable steps you can do right away.

LET'S GET STARTED!

Warming up

Like with any exercise, the correct clothing is key to staying comfortable. Clothes that are not too baggy but not uncomfortably tight – pretty much what most people dress like for the gym, is ideal – so, fitted leggings or shorts, and a top that's tight enough so it doesn't flap about and get in the way.

You will get very warm during the workouts, so if you're taking your workout outside add layers which can easily be removed as you warm up. Overheating is uncomfortable at best, dangerous at worst.

Sturdy shoes will prevent slipping or tripping up, and a hat and sunscreen in summer go without saying.

Keep a bottle of water nearby to stay hydrated – a screw top plastic bottle is better than a regular glass if you're outside as it won't break and won't spill if it falls over while resting on less even surfaces than indoors.

Everyone should do some warming up before exercising – it preps the muscles and joints for what is to come by activating your muscles, and a few mobility exercises will get your blood flowing and lubricate your joints.

If you're feeling really stiff or are new to exercise, warming up is extra important. Spending 3–5 minutes warming up is about right for most people.

Starting from the bottom and working up is a good way to remember to do each joint. Some good ideas include:

- **ankle rotations** – circle your feet 5 times each way, one foot at a time

- **knee swings** – standing on one leg and holding on to something for support, let one foot off the ground so that your knee is bent, and swing it gently to the front (like you want to return a football with your knee) and back again, repeat on the other leg

- **hip circles** – stand with your feet hip width apart and make a circle with your hips as wide as they will go, 5 times each way

- **shoulder circles** – with your arms by your side, circle your shoulders backwards then forwards, 5 times each way

- **arm circles** – swing your arms right over your head and round again, 5 times forwards then 5 times backwards

- **elbow and wrist circles** – circle each joint 5 times each way

- **finger wiggles** – wriggle your fingers like you're playing the piano. The fingers aren't often used in conventional exercise but you'll most likely use them quite a lot when gardening, writing, and in most daily tasks

- **jogging on the spot** and **jumping jack**s get your heart and lungs working a little

- a few body weight **squats** and **knees down press ups** are good for mobilising your knee, elbow and shoulder joints.

The workout

The best exercise is the one you enjoy and the one you stick to. Consistency, that is keeping to a realistic schedule and very rarely missing a workout, is more important than what you actually choose to do for that workout. That being said, most women already have enough on their plate with work, children, organising a wedding, ... ! So anything that can be done in as short a time as possible while still making progress makes sense. I prefer High Intensity Interval Training (HIIT) for this reason, and is what I coach on my The Fit Mum Formula 'BodyBack' programme. Do the following routine 3–5 times a week, with at least a day's rest between each workout, and walk as much as you can, preferably at least 30 minutes a day, to help reduce stress, burn more calories and help your muscles recover faster from your HIIT workouts.

Using this workout template targets the three areas of your body – upper body, legs, core and also some cardio, meaning you get a full body workout – always begin with a warm up (see the previous section).

Get a piece of paper, a scrap one will do. Divide it into 5 sections, these are your 5 'rounds'.

In each round, choose one exercise from each body part or exercise type; upper body, core, lower body, and cardio. If you want to keep it simple at first and just keep repeating the same exercises as round 1 for the other rounds that's fine. But the more exercise variety you do, the greater and more varied the benefits, so try and switch it up a bit, if not within the same workout, then for your next workout in a couple of days' time.

Set a countdown timer for 25 minutes. You will almost certainly have this function on your mobile phone, or else there are apps you can download.

Do as many as you can of each exercise for 1 minute each, then once you have done all four exercises (4 minutes) rest for 1 minute, then move on to round 2.

If you're new to this type of exercise you might not manage many of each at first – you'll likely need to pause between press ups, for example. But you'll progress quickly with consistency.

The idea of HIIT is that you work as hard as you can – push yourself hard (but stop if you feel pain instead of just tired muscles) and make sure you rest properly between rounds.

Video demonstrations for all the exercises listed can be found on this URL:

https://www.youtube.com/list?list=PL60XJ4XEa8wwpefMXKgdYgQtut9haz9BS)

	ROUND 1	ROUND 2	ROUND 3	ROUND 4	ROUND 5
UPPER BODY	e.g. Box press up				
CORE	e.g. Walking plank				
LOWER BODY	e.g. Reverse lunges				
CARDIO	e.g. Mountain climbers				

UPPER BODY EXERCISES

Your upper body – arms, back and shoulders – are more visible than other body parts, especially during the warmer summer months, so from an aesthetic point of view everyone likes to have a nice set of arms to show off when the woolly jumpers get removed.

From a functional point of view having a strong upper body makes life a lot easier. Carrying shopping bags, lifting children and clearing heavy items from the attic are all much easier and safer if you have the muscles to support your joints and back. Injuries caused by lifting things heavier than you can safely manage mean you could be off exercise for months while you recover, which is definitely a setback in the long run.

Doing upper body exercises, even without weights, will help give you the strength and stability to carry out heavy tasks without tiring out so fast, risking injury, or having to ask for help each time something needs moving!

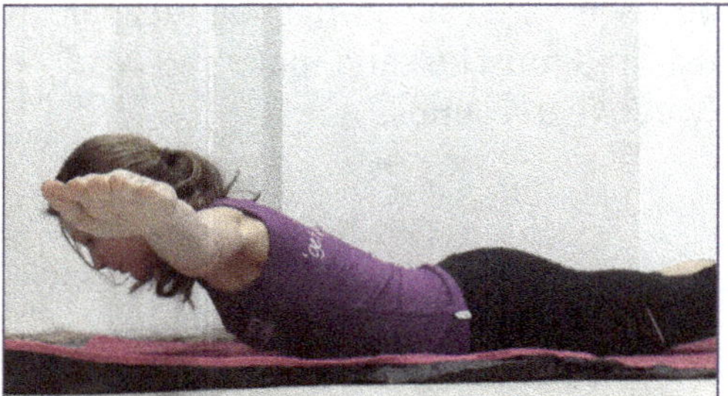

Batmans
Lie on your front with your legs straight out behind you and arms stretched out to the side (like batman flying). Raise your upper body and arms from the hips, as well as your feet, and pulse, trying not to drop your arms or feet to the ground, and keeping your neck straight.

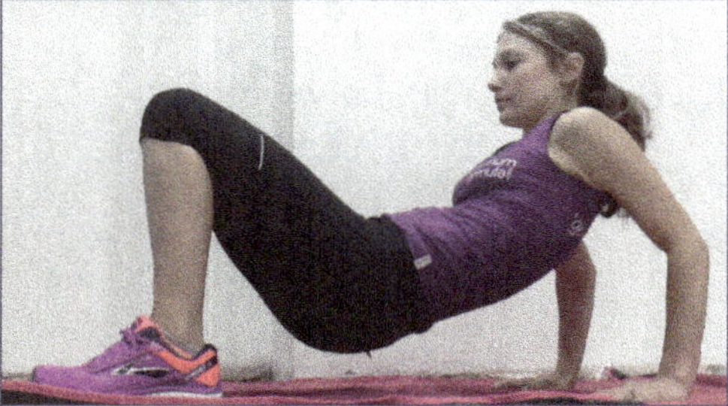

Tricep dips
Place your hands shoulder width apart on a step or bench behind you (or just on the floor), and put your legs bent out in front, facing up. Bend your elbows, pointing them backwards, to lower your body, then straighten the elbows to raise your body up. Repeat.

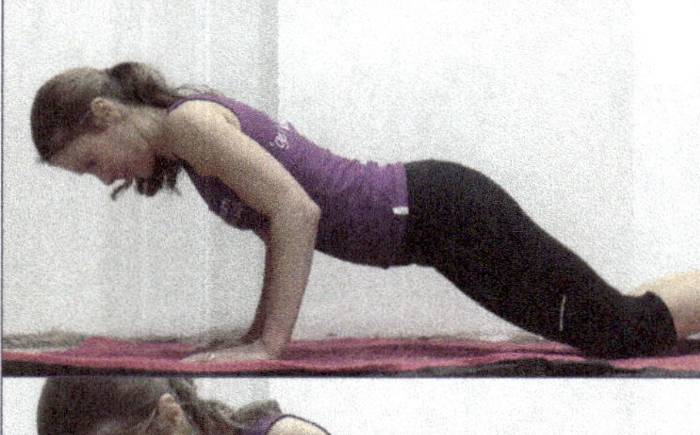

Press ups and variations
Lie on the floor facing down and lift your body up so it is supported by your hands and feet, shoulder width apart. If a full press up is too much, put your knees on the ground. Lower your body until your chest nears the floor, pointing your elbows back or to the side (both are acceptable) then return to the starting position.

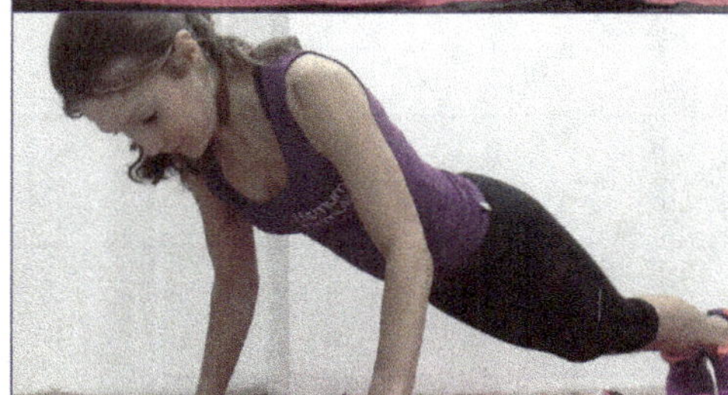

Walking push ups
Start with a regular push up, then move your hands a few inches to the left (to an 11 o'clock position) while keeping your feet still, and do another push up. Move hands left further (10 o'clock) then press up again. Reverse inwards then repeat on the right.

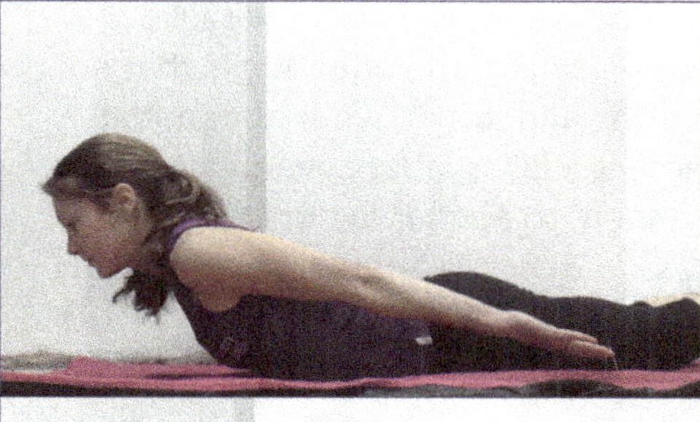

Back extension

Lie on your front with arms by your side and nose to the floor. Lift your shoulders and feet off the floor so that you are resting on your torso, hold for as long as possible, lower, then repeat.

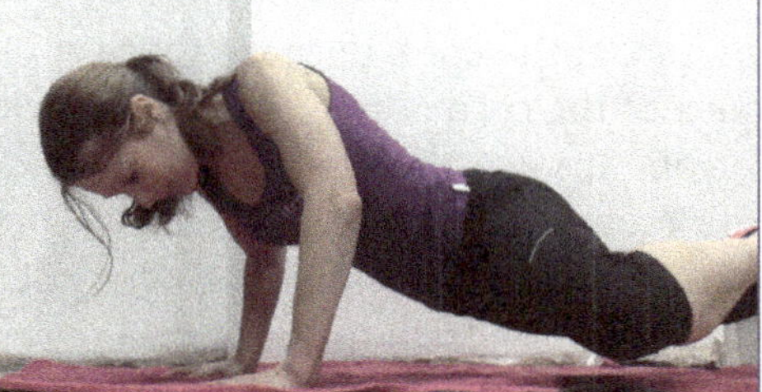

Spiderman push up

As you do a regular push up, bring on knee up toward your hip as you lower, so that your leg is bent and looking like Spiderman climbing a wall! Then take it back to the starting position as you return to straight arms.

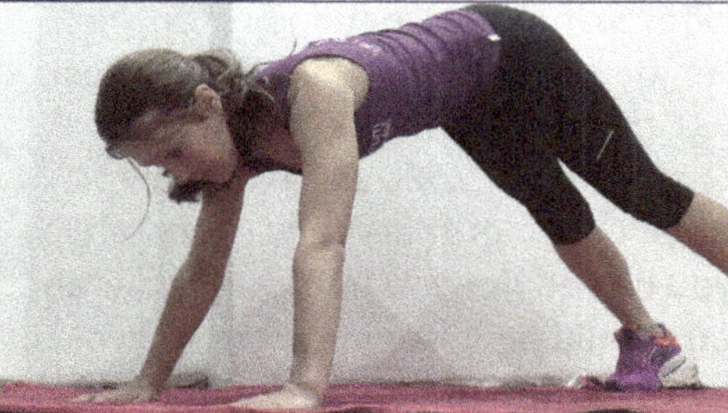

V press up

Rest on your hands and feet with bottom pointing in the air, so you make an upturned 'V' shape. Bend elbows outwards to lower your upper body toward the floor, then straighten to raise up again.

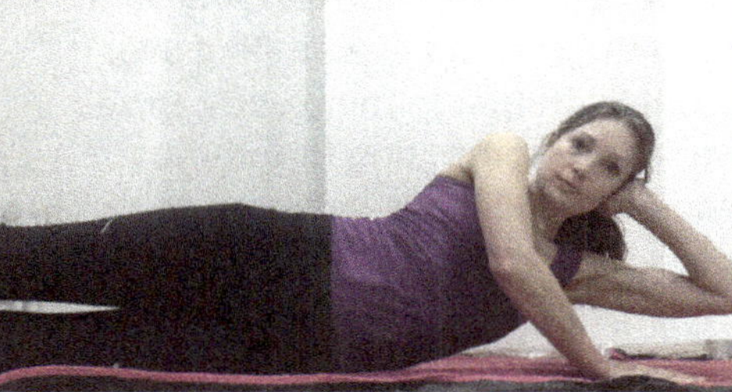

Side lying tricep dip

Lie on your side, legs outstretched in a straight line. Bring your underside arm up and use your hand to support your head (like you were sleeping) and place your upper arm hand on the floor in front of your chest. Push on your upper arm to raise your upper body off the floor, then lower.

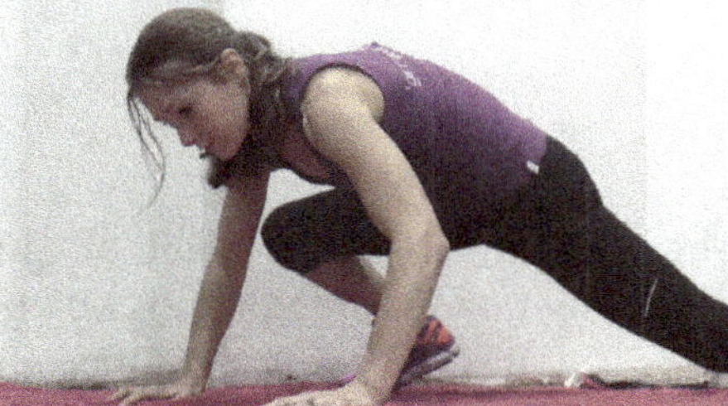

Bear crawl

Moving forwards on your hands and feet, as if you were walking but at the same time bent over, using your hands to 'walk' too.

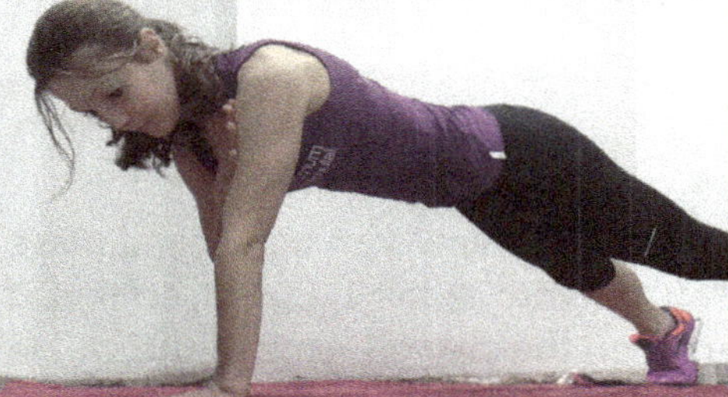

Shoulder taps

Begin in a press up position. Lift one hand and tap the opposite shoulder, then place back on the floor. Repeat with the other hand. Do this ongoing as fast as you can while not wobbling or letting your body sag in the middle.

CORE EXERCISES

It's a misunderstanding that you need to do hundreds of targeted core exercises, like sit ups and crunches, to get abs. In fact, most exercises, especially full body compound exercises that use more than one muscle group, will use the core to some extent to stabilise the body, keep you in position and prevent you from toppling over! If it's visible abs you're after, diet plays a more important part as you'll need to reduce body fat levels through eating a caloric deficit to be able to see the six-pack you've developed. That being said, core exercises do work, and will help build up the six-pack muscles, as well as the surrounding and back muscles that help stabilise your spine and prevent back injuries.

What are abs?

Abs is short for abdominal muscles, comprised of the transverse abdominis, internal and external obliques and rectus abdominis. These work together with all the muscles in your back to stabilise your spine and provide the necessary strength and flexibility to bend, stretch, rotate, push (an awkward and full shopping trolley), pull (a heavy door open), lift (a crying child) and carry (a suitcase).

What most gym-goers and exercise fans (or newbies) are actually referring to is the visibility of the rectus abdominis muscles, which form 'sections' down the front of the torso, and are more commonly known as the six-pack.

Why don't fit people always have a six-pack? Because the other side of the equation is that no matter how strong and 'toned' your abdominal muscles, if there is a layer of fat covering them they won't be seen, so aiming to burn fat through achieving a calorie deficit is also necessary if you want your six-pack to be visible.

How to work your abs

Also known as part of the core, because these muscles are part of the core of our body, past advice for improving your abs was to do endless exercises that used these muscles in isolation – sit ups, crunches, and twists in numbers higher than most people have the attention span to count.

Unfortunately (or fortunately, depending on whether you enjoy sit ups or not!) it's not as clear cut as that. BUT the good (if not better) news is that you don't have to do 1,000 sit ups a day to see results either. Consider that many every day movements you do require you to engage your abs (or at least you should be engaging them to avoid over using other muscles and to prevent injuries) – bending down to pick things up, carrying your shopping in from the car, and even rolling over to get out of bed! With that in mind you can see that doing a variety of compound (multi-muscle) exercises are a better and more balanced route than endless crunches.

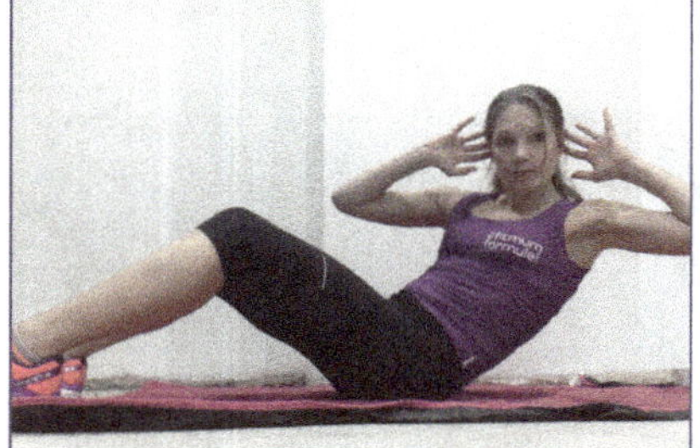

Oblique twists
Basically a sit up with a twist, targeting the muscles at the side of your waist. Lie on your back, knees bent and feet on the floor, hands behind your head. Lift your upper body and twist left so that your right elbow is pointing toward your left knee. Lower and repeat on the other side.

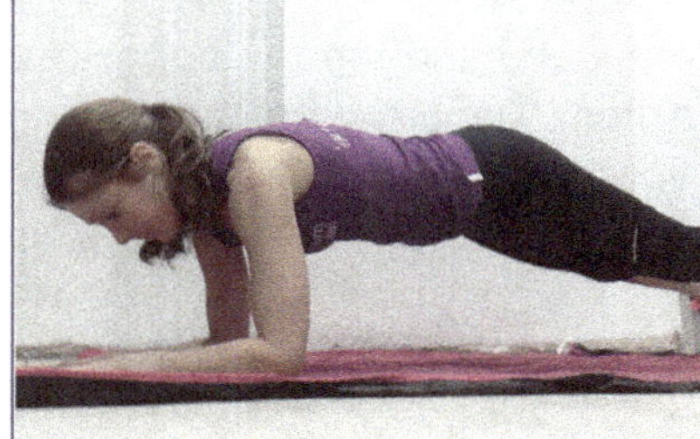

Plank
Lie on your front, legs out behind you, feet hip width apart, and place your hands under your shoulders. Raise your entire body up, so that it stays straight, keeping your forearms on the ground. Engage the whole body, but especially the core, so that you don't sag in the middle.

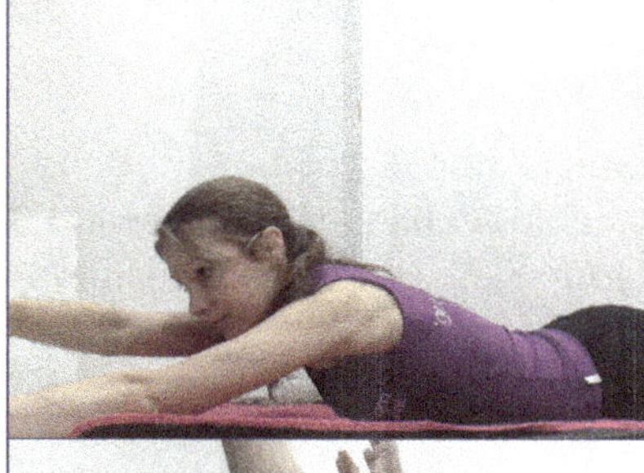

Swimmers

Lie on your front, legs straight behind you and arms stretched out front. Raise your arms and legs off the ground, keeping your neck aligned with your spine. Both arms and legs pulse at the same time but opposite sides, so one arm will be up while the other is down, hence the 'swimming' name.

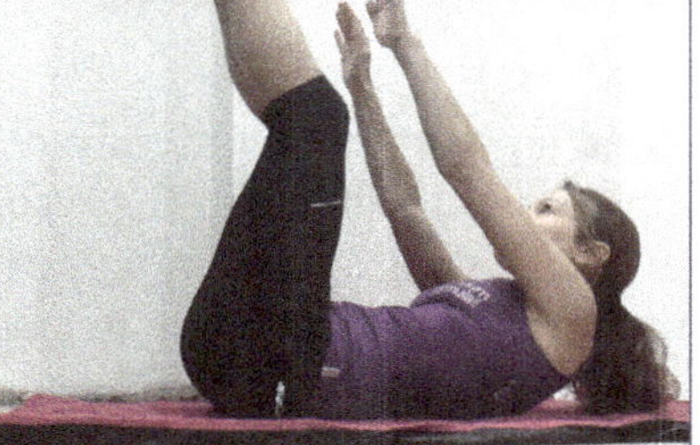

Reverse crunches

Lie on your back with your feet pointing to the ceiling and knees slightly bent. Use your core muscles to lift the lower half of your torso off the ground, raising your legs higher in the process, lower, and repeat.

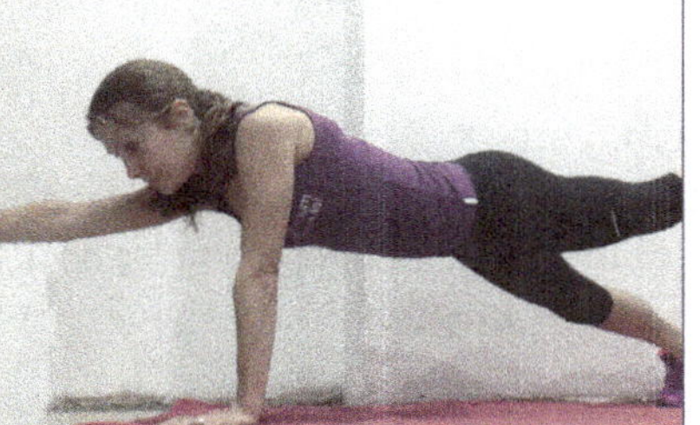

Superman plank

Begin in a plank position resting on your hands, then stretch your right hand forward and lift your left leg off the floor. Hold for 30 seconds then switch hands and legs.

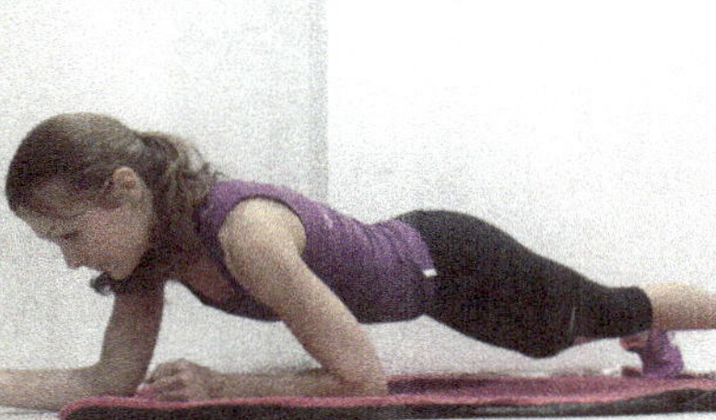

Walking plank

Begin in a plank position resting on your forearms. Inch forward by moving one arm and foot forward at a time, all the while keeping your body straight and strong.

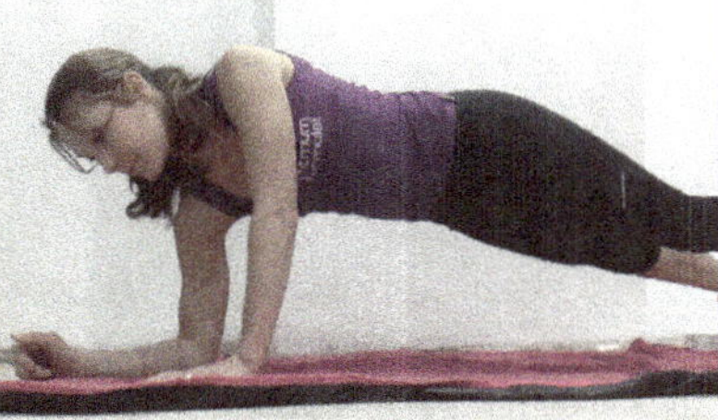

Plank with weight transfer

Assume a plank position with forearms on the ground. Step up on to one hand then the other, then return one forearm after the other to the ground in a walking rhythm.

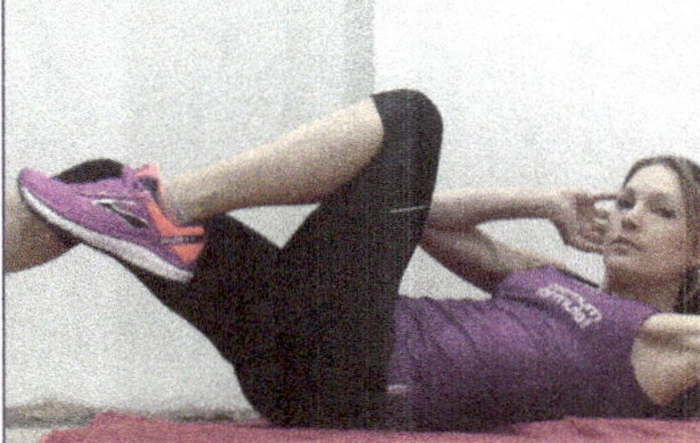

Bicycles

Lie on your back with your hands behind your ears. Lift your feet off the floor and bend your knees to 90°. Move your legs in a cycling motion, reaching the opposite elbow forward to the knee as each knee comes toward your head.

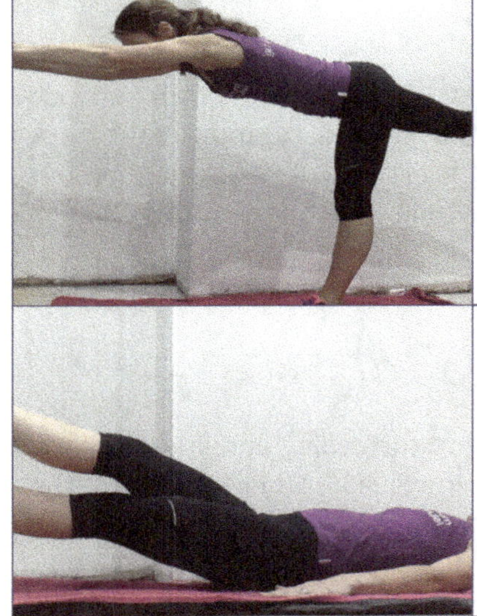

Forward balance

Stand in a neutral position with arms straight above your head. Bend forward lifting your right leg straight out behind while leaning forward, keeping your back straight and arms by your ears. Hold for 30 seconds then return to starting position and switch legs.

Horizontal scissor kicks

Lie on your back with arms by your side and legs stretched out in front of you. Raise your feet a few inches off the ground and widen them so there's a foot space between your ankles. Move your feet toward each other so that one foot passes over the other, then return and repeat, but with the other foot passing on top.

LOWER BODY EXERCISES

The leg muscles are the largest in the body, meaning that when you use them, you get a lot of bang for your buck in terms of calorie burning, muscle building and other benefits of exercise, like improving insulin sensitivity (important in keeping blood sugar levels healthy and preventing diabetes). Having strong legs will help prevent injuries due to joint instability – not enough muscle to keep joints aligned properly when moving, especially under intense loads when exercising. Gluteal muscles in particular play a big role in posture and back health, meaning you're less likely to have backache if you have a strong and pert bottom!

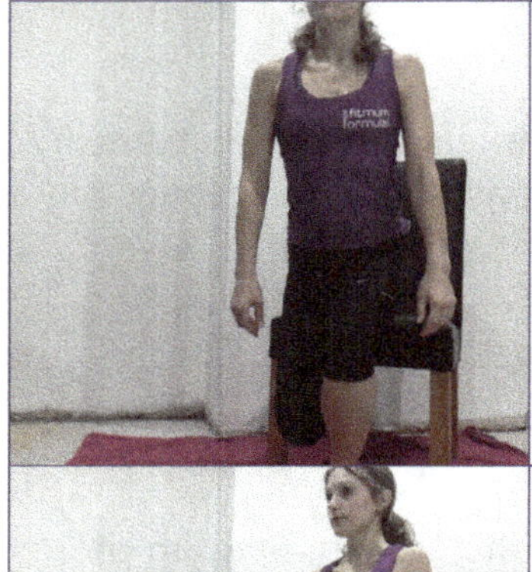

Bulgarian split squats

Stand in front of a stable chair and place one foot on the chair behind you. Bend your standing leg, keeping your knee over your foot (move your standing food forward if necessary), and try and get your back knee as low to the ground as possible. Straighten your front leg to stand, repeat. Switch legs after 30 seconds.

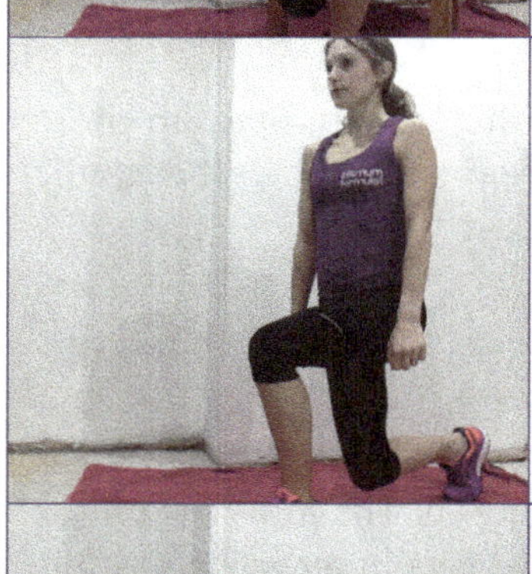

Reverse lunge

Start feet hip width apart. Squeeze the glutes and step backwards with one leg into a lunge position, landing with the front knee positioned over the front foot and back knee close to the ground. Step forward to starting position. Alternate legs or do 30 seconds on each leg.

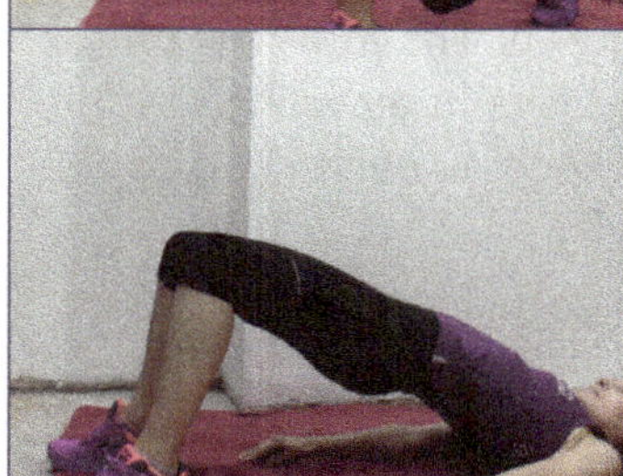

Glute bridge

Lie on your back with knees bent to 45 degrees and feet flat on the floor, hands by your side. Lift your hips high enough to create a straight line from your torso along the front thighs to your knees. Lower, and repeat.

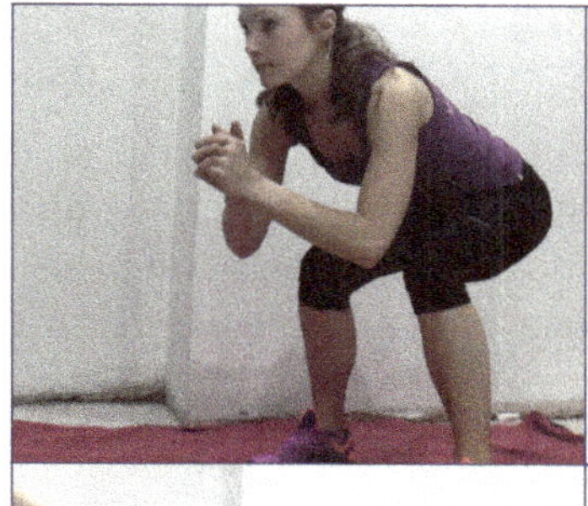

Squats
Stand with your head facing forward and place your feet slightly wider than shoulder-width apart. Sit back and down like you're sitting into a chair, lowering your thighs as parallel to the floor as possible, with your knees over your ankles. Return to standing.

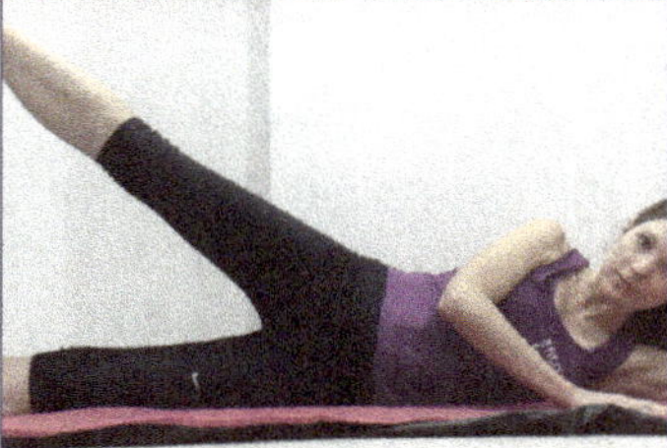

Abductor raise
Lie on your side with your legs outstretched in a straight line. Raise your top leg, keeping it straight, so that your foot is pointing to the corner of the room. Lower in a controlled manner and repeat.

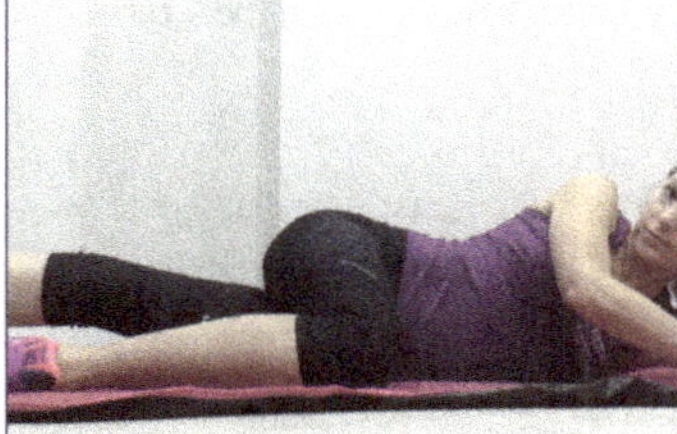

Adductors raise
Lie on your side with your legs outstretched in a straight line. Take your top knee and bring it forward to rest on the floor in front of your lower leg. Raise your underside leg, keeping it straight, so that your foot is pointing to the corner of the room. Lower in a controlled manner and repeat.

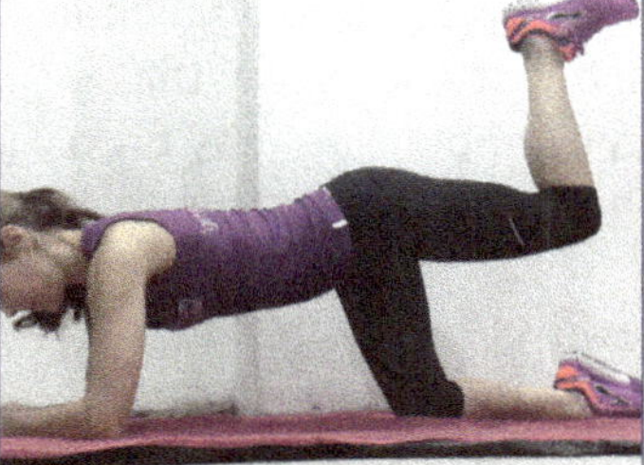

Bent leg donkey kicks
Start on all fours, resting on your hands and knees, making a box shape under your torso. Lift one leg up behind you so that your knee points back and foot to the ceiling, and pulse.

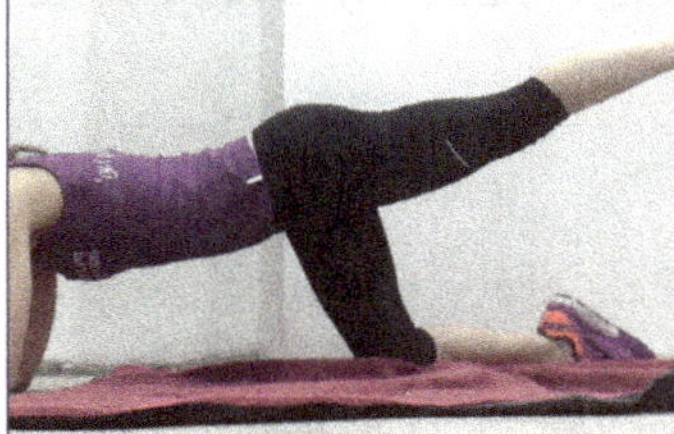

Straight leg donkey kicks
Start on all fours, resting on your hands and knees, making a box shape under your torso. Lift one foot out straight behind you so that your leg is straight out pointing backwards, and pulse.

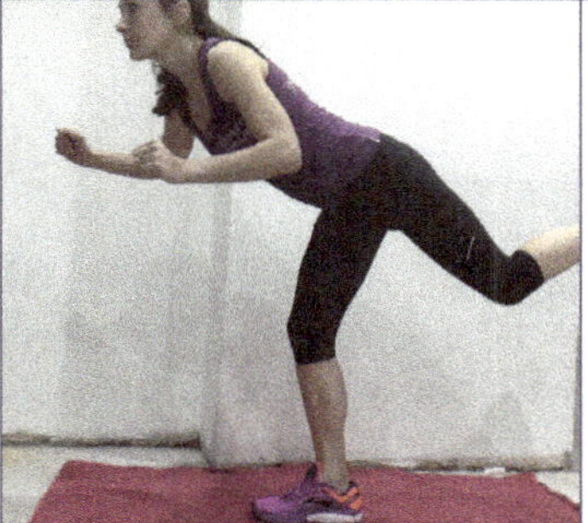

Kickbacks
Stand with feet a little wider than hip width apart. Squat down, then as you straighten up kick one leg forcefully out back behind you (make sure there's nothing in the way!). Bring your foot back down and squat again as you do so, then raise out and kick back with the other leg.

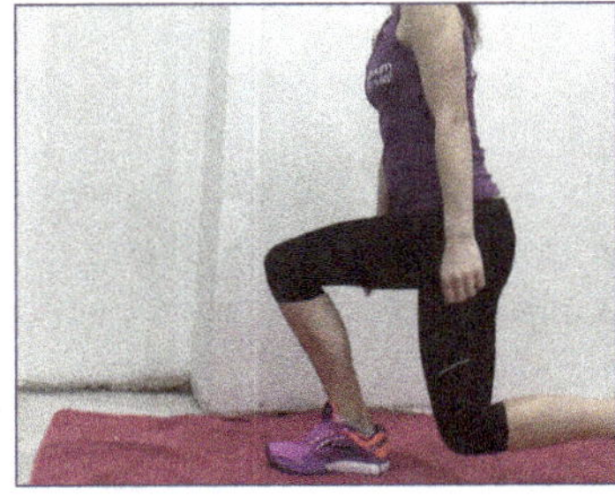

Walking lunges
From a standing position step forward into a lunge. Bring your back leg up forwards, toward your body, but rather than put it down step straight into the next lunge. When you run out of space simply turn around and carry on.

CARDIO EXERCISES

Cardiovascular exercise is good for getting your heart rate up, working your lungs and improving stamina. But you don't have to leave the house for a run or spend hours on the treadmill. As long as you can feel your body temperature rising, your heart beating faster and your lungs working harder to get air in, you'll be getting all the benefits of cardiovascular exercise from the comfort of your home or garden.

I'm not a fan of steady state cardio for fat loss. It's great for working your lungs and heart, and some people love it for stress relief (not me I might add!), but you get very little bang for your buck when it comes to weight loss.

Unlike resistance training (bodyweight, like the BodyBack workouts or system in this book, or traditional weight training), the calorie burning stops as soon as you stop jogging. With intense resistance workouts you get this magic 'afterburn', where you keep burning calories for hours after you finish your workout!

Longer bouts of cardio also produce more stress hormones (that encourage fat storing and muscle loss, exactly the opposite of what we want to happen), and make you feel hungry, especially if you're doing it in cold weather. This might make sense since you're just burnt off a load of calories, but studies show that for many people the hunger induced is disproportionate to the calories burnt — as an example, you may burn 200 calories, but are then really hungry for 300 calories of extra food, and since hunger is hard to ignore, you can see why it doesn't do you many favours if weight loss is your goal.

There is a caveat, and that is that short, intense bursts of cardio exercise, like sprint intervals or HIIT, are great for the lungs and heart and improve your overall fitness levels, insulin sensitivity (so your body handles carbohydrates more effectively), and fat loss, without the less desirable effects of slow, steady state cardio.

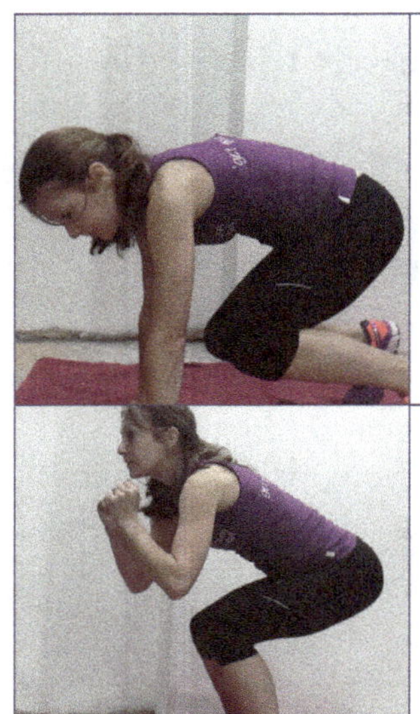

Burpees
A series of smaller movements which create one exercise move when done quickly in sequence. Start in a neutral standing position. Crouch down and put your hands on the floor in front of you. Jump backwards to a push up position and do a push up. Jump forward, placing your feet behind your hands, before jumping in the air and landing and going straight into the next burpee if you can.

Tuck jumps
Stand in a neutral position. Bend the knees then jump with enough force and power to bring your knees as high as you can to your chest before landing, bending the knees slightly as you land. Repeat.

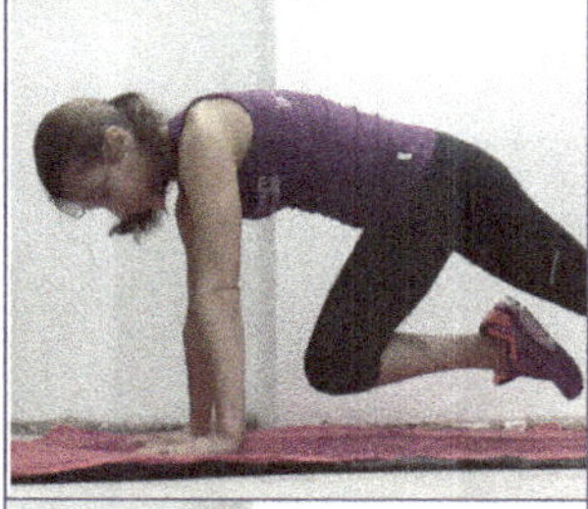

Mountain climbers

Place both hands and feet on the floor, facing down, as if in the starting position for a race but both feet are back behind you. 'Run' by bringing one knee forward at a time at speed, then quickly switching to the other knee coming forward.

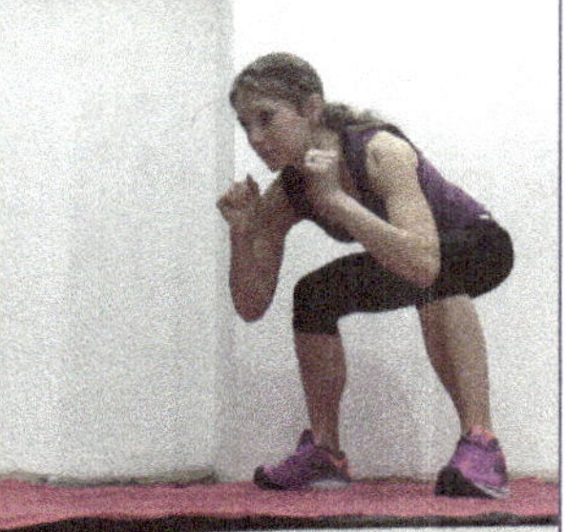

Jump squats

Stand looking straight ahead with your feet slightly wider than hip width apart. Move your hips back and down like you're sitting on a chair, lowering your thighs as parallel to the floor as possible, with your knees over your ankles. Drive your feet into the floor, propelling yourself into a jump, then land bending your knees back into the squat position before quickly driving back up into another jump.

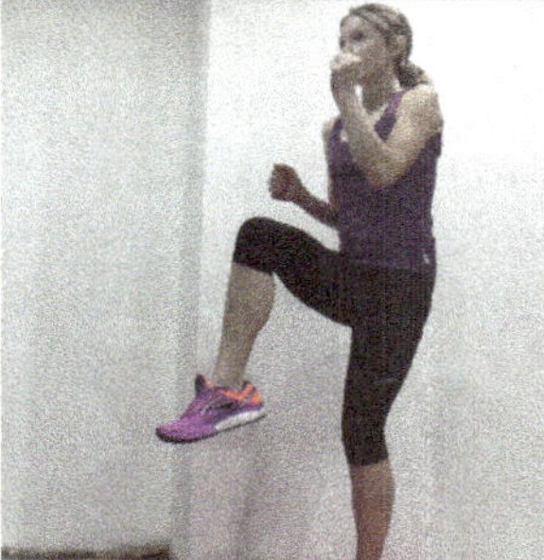

High knee sprints

Jogging on the spot, but bringing your knees up as high as you can, as fast as you can.

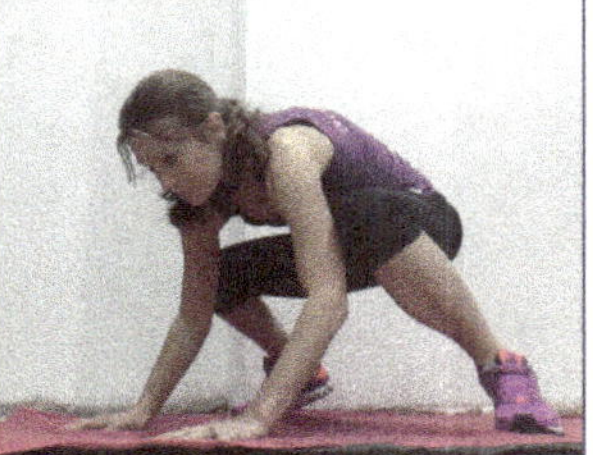

Plank to frogger jumps

Start in a plank position but with hands on the ground. Jump both feet forwards at the same time so that they land outside of your hands, like a frog sits, keeping your hands on the floor. Jump back to plank position, and repeat.

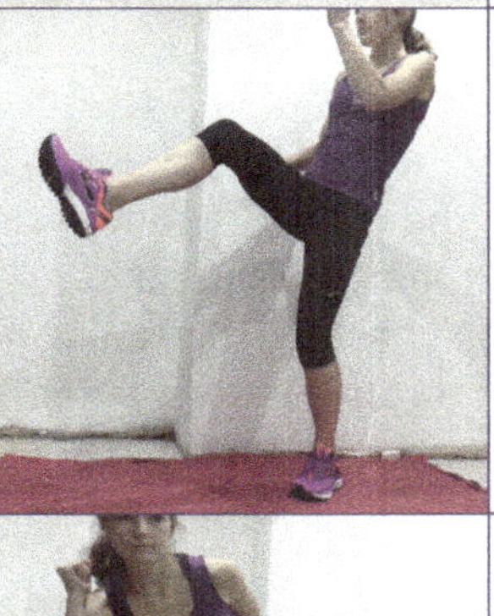

Switch kicks alternate legs

Do a high kick, akin to what you see in karate (make sure there's nothing in the way!). Jump on to the leg that's just kicked while bringing up the standing leg, so you're 'switching' between kicking legs.

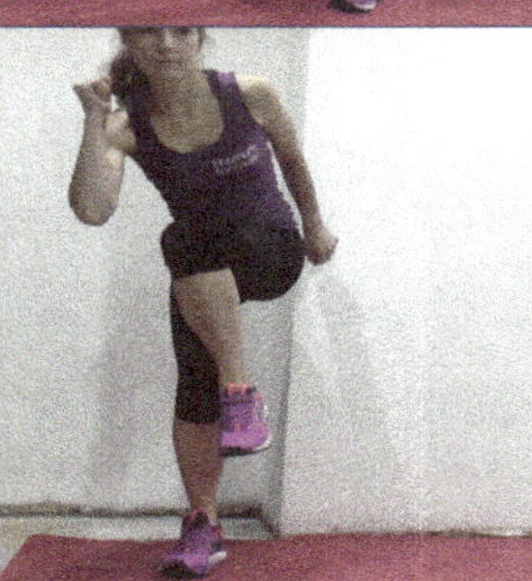

Heisman run

Side to side running with a knee lift at each side. From standing, step right, then bring the left leg to meet the right one quickly, step right again and bring your left knee up to your chest. From here step left into the next 'run' in the other direction.

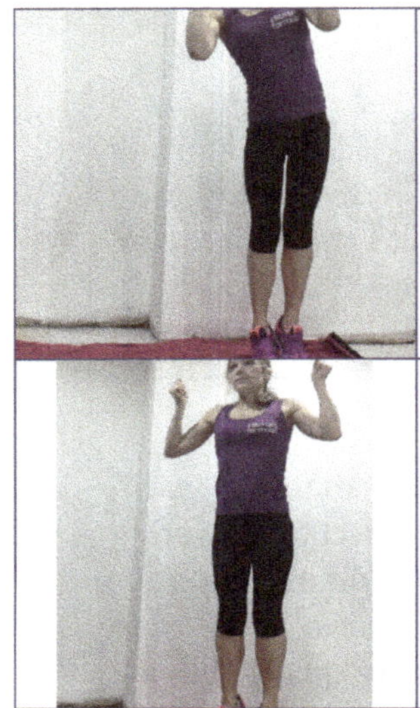

Ski jumps
Stand straight upright with both feet together. Jump from side to side in a skiing motion, keeping feet and knees together.

Double jump rope skips
Skip with an imaginary skipping rope (or real if you have one – make sure there's nothing in the way), jumping high and swinging your arms fast as if you were trying to get the rope over twice before landing.

COOLING DOWN

Spend a couple of minutes when you've finished stretching each muscle and holding for about 20–30 seconds so you're less likely to feel stiff the next day, and make sure you have a good drink to replenish any water lost through sweating.

Inner thighs

Sit with your back straight and legs bent, feet on the floor close to your buttocks, knees pointing to the ceiling. Lower your knees outwards toward the floor until you feel a strong resistance, and hold.

Calves

From standing, take a big step forward with one foot and bend your front leg, keeping the back leg straight, so that you feel the stretch down the back of your lower leg. Hold.

Quads

Lie on your side, legs straight out, knees together. Take hold of the foot on your upper leg and pull it toward your buttocks, keeping your knees together; you should feel the stretch down the front of your thigh.

Hip flexors

An easily missed stretch, hip flexors are just lower than your hip bones, connecting the front of your hips to your thighs. Step forward into a low lunge, and move your hips forward while keeping the back foot on the ground, until you feel a stretch just under your hip bones, but above the front of your thighs.

Hamstrings

Lie on your back with your legs bent and feet on the floor (sit up starting position). Take hold of one thigh or calf and point the leg toward the ceiling, foot flexed with your heel pointing upwards. Pull your leg toward you until you feel a stretch in the back of your thigh and hold.

Glutes

Lie on your back, bring your knees into your chest. Turn one knee outwards and rest that foot on the opposite thigh. Put a little pressure on the turned out thigh until you feel the stretch in your buttock, and hold.

Chest

Stand with your arms stretched behind you and interlink your fingers. Push your hands backwards so that you feel the stretch across your chest.

Triceps/shoulders

Take one arm overhead, bend at the elbow joint, and extend your hand down the centre of your back, gently pulling the elbow with the opposite hand. Take the same arm across the chest, gently pulling at the elbow joint, to extend through the shoulder. Switch arms.

Core/back

On all fours, round out your back (like an angry cat), and then invert it, making a C-shape with your spine.

Other ideas

Low intensity walking, foam rolling and massage are all awesome ways to help recover from intense exercise, as well as reduce stress, aid circulation and improve general wellbeing.

FOOD

THE BASICS START HERE

The best foods for weight loss just happen to be the ones that also allow you to feel satisfied and bouncing with energy, while giving you sparkling eyes, glowing skin and glossy hair. I don't prescribe meal plans as most people find them too complicated to stick to when life is busy enough, however, following this set of guidelines 90% of the time (leaving 10% for treats) is a pretty reliable way to improve your waistline as well as your health in almost every way.

I appreciate you're a busy Mum and won't be reading this book cover to cover in one sitting. So by drip-feeding actionable steps there's no reason you can't start eating in ways that will get you closer to your goals, today. Here are the fundamentals of a healthy weight loss diet:

- fill half your plate with vegetables or salad before you add other foods

- if you're extra hungry and want second helpings, go for more salad or vegetables first

- make at least ¼ to 1/3 of your plate a whole protein source – chicken, beef, salmon, etc. – as opposed to processed options like fishcakes or sausages, which are usually lower quality and bulked up with other, less nutritious ingredients. If you want, say, fishcakes, which usually contain quite a large proportion of potato, have them and omit any extra potatoes, since you're already getting some; quiche is another example, the starchy carbs are in the pastry

- don't omit carbohydrates, you'll only crave them more, but keep them to ¼ of your plate or less to avoid blood sugar fluctuations (and cravings)

- don't omit fat; it's essential to health, makes your skin and hair glow, and makes meals tastier and more satiating. Avocados, coconut products, olives and oily fish are excellent, but there's nothing wrong with fattier cuts of meat, like lamb or beef, either, so long as it doesn't contribute to eating more calories than you need. Likewise nuts and nut butters are very nutritious, but are easy to overeat, so stick to 1 tbsp. of nut butter or 2 tbsp. nuts as a serving

- experiment with breakfasts other than toast or cereal. Proteins like eggs, protein shakes, pancakes made with flours like quinoa or buckwheat flour, or Greek yoghurt are much more nutritious and satiating.

Here's an example of a Sunday roast my Mum cooked. Any meal can be made healthier simply by adjusting the portions of each food group.

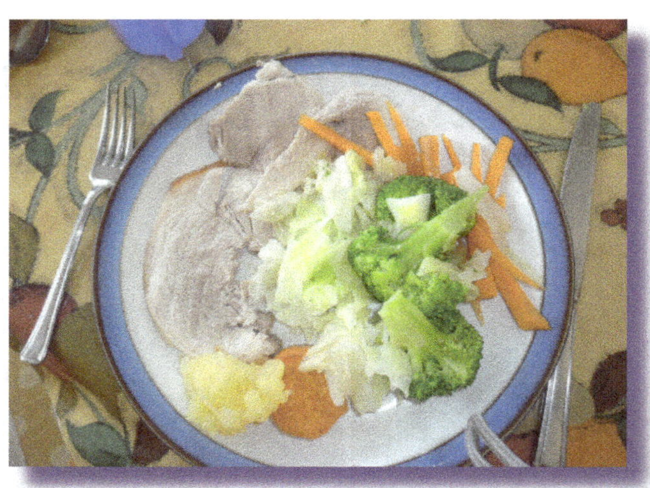

EXAMPLE MEAL PLAN

About using this example meal plan

These are very simplistic list of ideas so as not to overcomplicate things, especially when you first join the programme and this way of eating is new to you. But, as you get used to choosing the foods that put you into a fat burning state, you will find the confidence to branch out and create your own combinations.

Try to vary your choices as much as possible, for example, if you have eggs for breakfast then have something different at lunch and for your evening meal, this way you will benefit from the largest range of nutrients.

Fresh food is preferred over convenience foods, but I'd rather you did what works for you and stick with it, rather than dictating a regime which is too hard to sustain.

Don't worry if you have leftovers, put them in the fridge to add to meals over the next few days. You can even mix and match according to whatever you have leftover – a platter of various cooked meats with a small mix of cooked rice, beans and lentils with your salad, for example, to avoid wastage. Just make sure you stick to the recommended portions. Any meal can work following your plate layout (including in restaurants), for instance, steak, jacket potato and salad; half a plate of veg or salad, 1/3 protein, and the rest a healthy starchy carb, with a little bit of fat if your protein is very lean (such as steamed white fish or baked skinless chicken).

When you are in a hurry, the cupboards are bare, or you need to grab something on the go, good quality protein powders and bars are much better than most convenience foods, and are certainly better than skipping a meal, or junk meals and snacks. While we would always advocate using real food ideally, it doesn't hurt to have a tub on standby for those 'too busy' times! They also work well to increase the protein content in some recipes and to turn a tasty and convenient smoothie into a satisfying meal or snack.

How to segment your portions – a starter guide!

You can make any meal using whatever you fancy (within reason) or have to hand, so long as it is in the right proportions. Note that due to our individual genetic make-up and lifestyle, the ideal balance will vary from person to person, and even change for an individual over time, but this is a good place to start before you tweak it to work better for you. Use this plate as a guide when serving yourself in any meal situation.

It is no coincidence that there are seven options for each 'meal' here, enough for something different to have each day. This is a very simplistic list of ideas so as not to overcomplicate things, especially when you first join the programme and this way of eating is new to you. But as you get used to choosing the foods that put you into a fat burning state you will find the confidence to branch out and create your own combinations.

Try to vary your choices as much as possible, for example if you have eggs for breakfast then have something different at lunch and for your evening meal; this way you will benefit from the largest range of nutrients. Fresh food is preferred over convenience foods, but we'd rather you did what works for you and stick with it, rather than dictating a regime which is too hard to sustain.

BREAKFAST

- pancakes: whisk one egg with 25g oat bran, 1 tsp. baking powder, 1 scoop (25g) protein powder and a little milk, to make a pancake batter. Fry using spray oil or a little coconut oil. Top with extra fruit

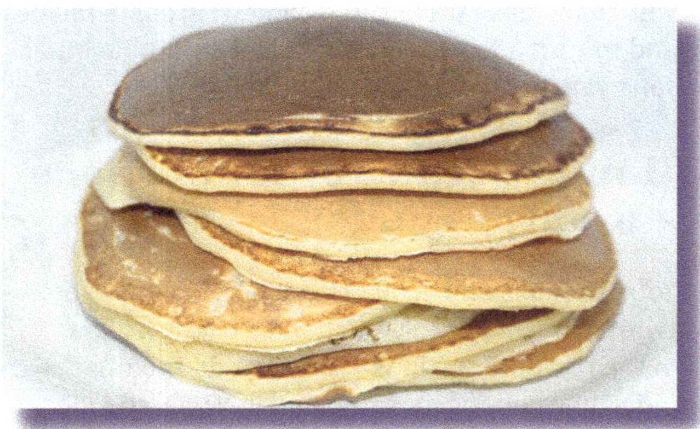

- scrambled eggs or an omelette: 4 egg whites or 2 whole eggs + unlimited vegetables (or a portion of fruit) + 1 small slice high fibre or rye bread

- 35g (dry weight) oatbran or whole oats cooked with water (sweeten with stevia if you like) or milk, plus 100g fat free Greek yoghurt + a piece of fruit

- 200g fat free Greek yoghurt + fruit

- 1 slice high fibre or rye bread with 2 tbsp. nut butter or 50g low fat cheese (e.g. cottage or cream cheese) + a portion of fruit

- 35g (dry weight) oatbran or whole oats made with hot water or milk and a scoop of protein powder + fruit

- protein smoothie or shake + a piece of fruit

MID-MORNING SNACK

- 1 portion of fruit or raw vegetables + a handful of nuts or 2 tbsp. nut butter

- 1 portion of raw vegetables + 150g cottage cheese

- 1 portion of fruit + 150 fat free Greek yoghurt

- 60g beef jerky + raw vegetables

- 1 hardboiled egg + raw vegetables

- 30g low sugar, high protein granola, without milk + fruit

- 1 flax seed crispbread spread with nut butter, reduced fat hummus, or cottage cheese + chopped fruit or veg

LUNCH

- 100g–150g lean protein with unlimited salad and 1 tbsp. dressing, topped with 1 tbsp. seeds (e.g. pumpkin or sunflower)

- half an avocado and either 150g prawns or 2 hardboiled eggs, on a large salad, with 2 tbsp. Greek yoghurt mixed with ketchup

- large salad + 100g–150g protein, dressed in 1 tbsp. dressing, 1 small whole-wheat tortilla

- chunky vegetable soup + 100g–150g protein (e.g. shredded turkey or chopped tempeh) + ½ high fibre bread roll

- scrambled eggs or an omelette: 4 egg whites or 2 whole eggs + 50g chopped meat or fish (or vegetarian protein) + unlimited vegetables or salad + 2–3 tbsp. kidney or baked beans

- 2 oatbran or flaxseed crispbreads + 50g reduced fat cheese or 150g cottage cheese + unlimited raw vegetables or salad

- 1 lean sausage or slice of lean back bacon, one egg (or an extra sausage or bacon slice), 1 slice high fibre bread or 100g baked beans + unlimited mushrooms and tomatoes

MID-AFTERNOON SNACK

- 1 portion of fruit or raw vegetables + a handful of nuts or 2 tbsp. nut butter

- low sugar nut, seed or protein bar

- 1 portion of fruit + 150g fat free Greek yoghurt

- 60g beef jerky + raw vegetables

- 1 hardboiled egg + raw vegetables

- 50g low sugar, high protein granola, without milk + fruit

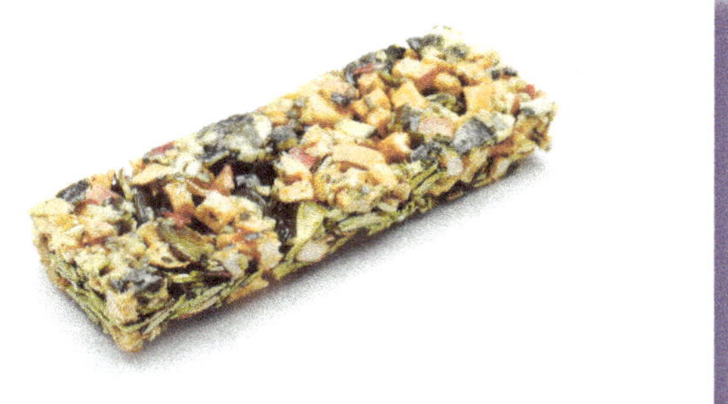

- chocolate-avocado pudding: mash ½ an avocado with 20g cocoa powder, 2 tsp. chocolate protein powder (optional) and 2 tsp. granulated stevia

EVENING MEAL

- stir fry 100g–150 g protein of your choice with 3 heaped tbsp. cooked wholegrain rice and unlimited vegetables, and some ground ginger, garlic, chilli, and soy sauce, to taste

- large salad with 100g–150g protein, dressed in 1 tbsp. vinaigrette + ½ a sweet potato

- chunky vegetable soup + 100g–150g protein (e.g. shredded turkey or chopped tofu) + 3 heaped tbsp. cooked lentils or quinoa, added to the soup

- scrambled eggs or an omelette: 4 egg whites or 2 whole eggs + 50g chopped meat or fish (or vegetarian protein) + 1–2 boiled new potatoes (unpeeled) + unlimited vegetables

- any protein based ready meal (e.g. meat or fish in cheese or tomato sauce, Quorn escalope, etc.), 3 heaped tbsp. cooked quinoa + unlimited vegetables

- chicken or beef burger, or 2 small Quorn burgers, topped with ½ a diced avocado and some tomato salsa, plus unlimited vegetables or salad

- 3 serving spoons of Bolognese sauce (around 200g), 3 heaped tbsp. wholemeal pasta + unlimited vegetables

EVENING SNACK

- 150ml milk and a small protein or nut, low sugar cookie

- 100g Greek yoghurt with 1 tsp. each of vanilla extract and stevia + some fruit

- 150ml milk + a small banana

- 30g protein granola with milk

- 200ml milk (with cocoa and stevia if you like) + 1 small portion of low sugar fruit (e.g. berries)

- small protein smoothie or shake

- 1 flaxseed cracker spread with nut butter, hummus or cottage cheese

Don't worry if you have leftovers, put them in the fridge to add to meals over the next few days. You can even mix and match according to whatever you have leftover – a mix of cooked rice, beans and lentils with your salad for example to avoid wastage. Just make sure you stick to your portion allowance.

WHAT TO EAT TO GET YOUR BODYBACK

Protein

Protein is the fire of your metabolism. It takes longer, and is harder, to digest than other food sources, so keeps your metabolism running at a higher speed for longer, uses more calories to digest, keeps you feeling full for longer, minimises cravings and keeps energy levels high but steady for longer. While not as low calorie as vegetables, it is very difficult to overeat on a diet high in protein and vegetables as they are so satiating. Imagine trying to eat 12 chicken breasts or ten fillet steaks with vegetables in one day! And that would still only just reach the 2,000 calories required by the average person to maintain a healthy weight. Protein is the second most abundant substance in the body after water, and eating enough of it will ensure adequate muscle tone, making you leaner, firmer and stronger, as well as playing a major role in immunity and body repair. Omega-3 rich proteins (oily fish, grass-fed meat and, to some extent, flax, chia and hemp seeds) are anti-inflammatory and have been shown to play a role in fat burning and, contrary to popular belief, saturated fats have no proven connection to heart disease and, in fact, play a vital role in body and brain functioning and in metabolism and satiety. Fatty protein sources are therefore absolutely fine, so long as they don't contribute to an excess in calories overall.

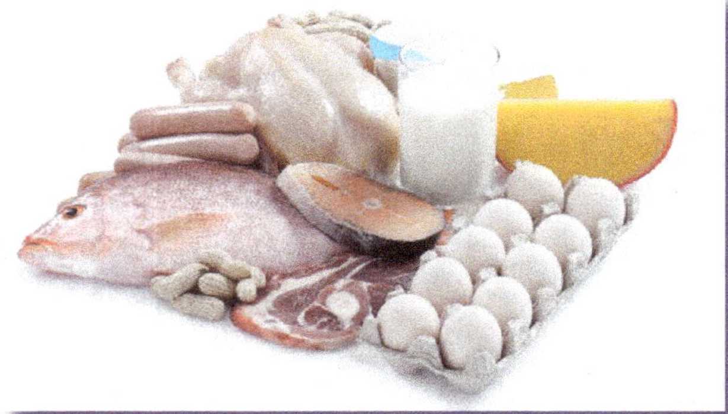

Animal products are the best sources of protein – chicken, beef, pork, turkey, lamb and game, as well as white and oily fish and shellfish. Incidentally grass-fed animals have higher levels of beneficial omega-3 fatty acids than corn-fed, so try to buy grass-fed meat where possible. Eggs are fantastic; the whites have more protein and are low calorie, so egg whites are a good way of eating more protein without extra calories, but the yolks are highly nutritious and whole eggs are a convenient and extremely healthy food to eat regularly. Free range, organic animal products are preferable but not essential; research has shown that hormones and antibiotics the animals are given may affect our health in numerous ways, but non-organic protein is still better than being deficient in protein. Try a farmer's market where small-scale producers can tell you exactly how their animals are reared and offer a good price. Beef jerky makes a good snack, and although wholefoods are always best, good quality protein powder/shakes (whey or a quality vegan blend with a good amino acid profile) and bars are much better than most convenience foods. Dried skimmed milk powder can be a convenient second choice option to protein shakes (it's higher in carbs and lower in protein, so use a quality protein powder where possible), if you run out of protein powder then try adding 25g dried skimmed milk to oatbran porridge, scrambled eggs, soups, etc. to bulk up the protein content.

Processed cheap meats, such as cheap sausages and salami, should be kept to a minimum as they are often high in salt, bulked up with added (unnecessary) ingredients, and lower in protein, plus, processing is a way of disguising the taste of poor quality meat. Good quality 'processed' meats, such as organic bacon and quality burgers and sausages are fine.

VEGETARIANS AND VEGANS

Just because meat is a feature part of the meal plan does not mean vegetarians and vegans can't also follow the programme, they just have to ensure protein consumption is adequate. There are many good vegetarian protein sources available. Plant based protein bars and shakes will probably feature more heavily in a vegan diet to ensure adequate protein intake and preserve muscle and good health. Eggs are high in protein, as is mycoprotein (Quorn), and also tofu, tempeh (fermented soy beans) and other soy products. Although soy is still better than beans and legumes as a protein choice, the oestrogenic effect it carries has been shown to negatively impact testosterone and thyroid hormones in some studies, so other protein based foods are preferable. The exception is tempeh, which is fermented, and fermented soy does not appear to have the same effects.

There is also protein to be found in other food groups; dairy products, such as cheese (especially low fat ones, such as fat free Greek yoghurt or cottage cheese) can be good sources. Nuts and seeds contain protein but are mostly fat. Beans, lentils and legumes also contain protein but are mostly starchy carbohydrate, so are categorised as such.

Fat

Fat does not make you fat. Fat is essential for brain function, nutrient absorption, skin and joint lubrication. It becomes a problem when consumed in high quantities as it is high in calories, or if the fats are of the unhealthy trans (hydrogenated) fat varieties, which are detrimental to health. Omega-3 fatty acids and another fat called CLA (found in meat and milk) act as metabolic messengers that increase fat burning, shrinking fat cells in both size and number, as well as building muscle. Saturated fats, contrary to popular belief, have no proven links to poor cardiovascular health and there is no need to avoid them.

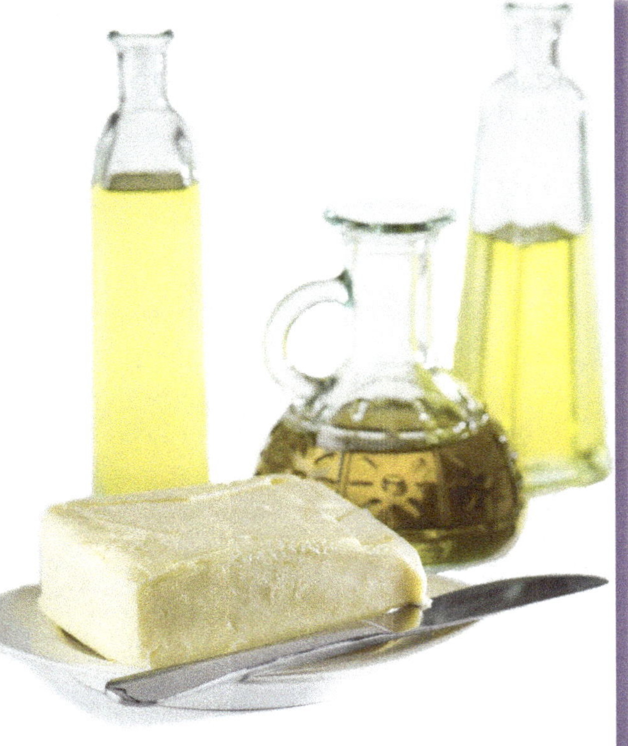

Monounsaturated (nuts, seeds, olives and olive oil, avocado) are great, as are polyunsaturated omegas -3, -6, and -9 (nuts, seeds and fish). However, we get plenty of -6 (excess omega-6 is actually thought to contribute heavily to inflammation) and our bodies make omega-9, so prioritise omega-3 fats from oily fish, flax, hemp and grass-fed meat. Have up to one handful of whole nuts or 2 tbsp. of no-added-sugar nut butter each day. Groundnuts can be used in place of flour in some recipes, as can coconut flour. Desiccated coconut and chopped nuts also feature in various healthy baking recipes, as does coconut oil, a medium chain triglyceride (MCT) saturated fat that is very nutritious, and is used more readily as energy than other fats. Flax seeds (meal or oil) are a source of omega-3 fatty acids for both vegetarians and meat eaters, and it is also low carb, high fibre, contains all 9 essential amino acids and is full of antioxidants. Vegetarians should take 1–3 tablespoons of flax oil per day, or alternatively hemp seeds or oil whose benefits are very similar. The downside of plant based omega-3s is that they need to be converted to a form the body prefers, and this conversion rate is low (under 10%) so you need to eat more of these than you would if you ate oily fish. Roughly 30%–40% of your daily calories should be from fat (about 60g–80g for an 1,800 calorie diet), however, as fat is dense in calories this won't look like a large amount in comparison to the calorie equivalent in high protein, fibre and water based foods.

Dairy

Dairy can be great or not so great, depending on your metabolic make up, the types of dairy you consume and in what quantities. Low fat, high protein dairy products (e.g. cottage cheese and Greek yoghurt) are lower in calories and are a good protein source. Higher fat dairy is fine, but just be mindful of the extra calories. Some people have difficulty digesting the lactose in milk due to allergies or intolerances. Calcium deficiency will not be an issue if you are eating plenty of other calcium rich foods, such as leafy green vegetables, almonds, oranges and bony fish, such as sardines.

One more useful tip. Dried skimmed milk powder can often be used in place of protein powder. They are, in general, higher in carbs and lower in protein and fat, so good whey (or vegan) protein powder is preferable. However, dried milk can be useful to have on standby to add a (neutral flavour) dose of protein to meals and recipes if you run out of protein powder.

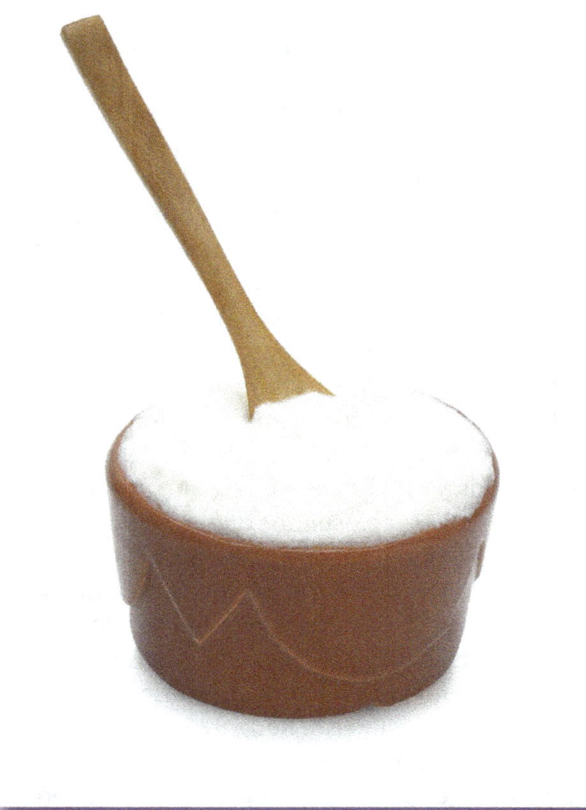

WHAT TO EAT

When it comes to dairy (if you have no intolerance or allergy, of course), low fat is not always the best as the vitamins in dairy products are fat soluble and are better absorbed in the presence of a little fat, so semi-skimmed and even whole milk are fine, as are full-fat yoghurts and cheese, and even cream in small amounts! A bigger problem is when they contribute to excess calories, though since fat is quite satiating you may find you are satisfied eating a smaller portion anyway. High protein dairy products, such as cottage cheese and Greek yoghurt, feature quite a lot in my meal plans and recipes as they contribute a good quantity of protein, so help reduce slow digestion and absorption and therefore make a good choice for vegetarians and meat eaters alike. However, fruit yoghurts that contain sugar and/or artificial sweeteners are not recommended, instead try flavouring yoghurt with fresh fruit, or spices such as cinnamon, plus some natural low calorie sweetener if you like (more on these below). Strong cheeses, such as parmesan are great; their flavour is strong enough that you only need a small amount.

If you think milk is disagreeing with you try cutting down for a while or switching to a nut milk – almond and drinking coconut milks are good if you've not got a nut allergy, and canned coconut milk is extremely nutritious – although high calorie due to the healthy fat content, so just be mindful of this. Rice milk isn't the best as it's derived from a carbohydrate source, and soy milk (like all unfermented soy products) mimics oestrogen so can encourage fat storage, as well as affecting the thyroid. Make sure you get calcium from non-dairy calcium rich foods, such as leafy greens, almonds, oranges and bony fish (e.g. sardines).

Vegetables and salad

High in fibre and water, vegetables are bulky (therefore filling) with very few calories. The fibre also contributes to satiation, as well as ensuring healthy, regular digestion, since you won't be getting as much fibre through starches and whole grains. Eat vegetables and salad vegetables in unlimited amounts. And the more variety you eat (aim for a whole rainbow of colours), the wider the variety of nutrients you will be getting, meaning that your whole body benefits more thoroughly. Lots of green vegetables are especially important when increasing protein consumption to ensure the body's pH does not become too acidic.

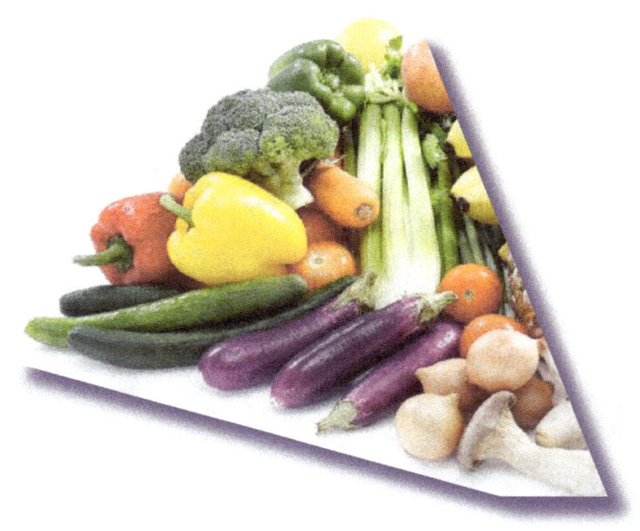

There are no rules against vegetables, eat all varieties freely and in unlimited amounts. The only thing you have to be aware of is that some things you may have thought were vegetables are actually higher in starchy carbohydrates and so should be eaten as such, rather than as a vegetable dish. These include white potatoes and sweet potatoes, Jerusalem artichokes, parsnips, broad beans and sweetcorn.

Fruit

Fruit is high in fibre and water, not to mention full of vitamins and antioxidants. The natural sugars present in fruit are a source of carbohydrate. Like vegetables they provide bulk without too many calories. Fresh is always best, but frozen can be useful to have on standby. Avoid dried fruit, which has had its water removed and therefore is more concentrated in sugar (unless in small amounts in recipes), and tinned, which has lost some of its nutrients due to being stored for a long time and can also be preserved in sugar syrup. Fruit juice is low fibre and high sugar (even freshly squeezed juices), so is not recommended, but pureeing the whole fruit (including skin) into smoothies is fine, though not as filling as whole fruit.

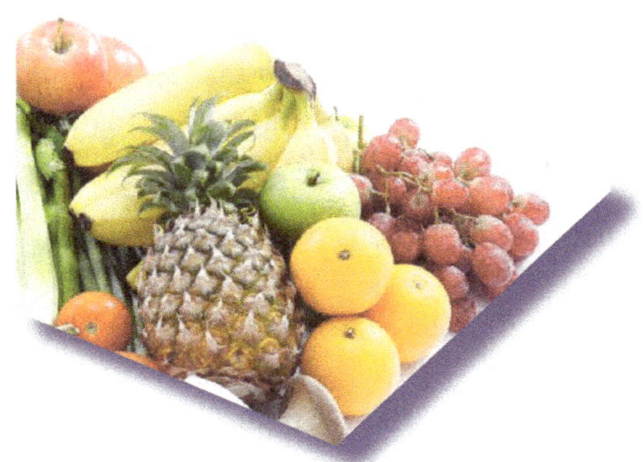

WHAT TO EAT

Overall, fruit is a great food and should be enjoyed freely. Fruits contain varying amounts of fructose (natural fruit sugar), tropical ones (mango, pineapple, bananas, papaya and watermelon and grapes, etc.) usually contain more. The high sugar content, albeit natural fructose, will raise blood sugar faster than low sugar fruits, such as apples, pears, lemons and limes, berries and cherries, and grapefruit, so eating large amounts of high sugar fruits is not a good idea, though they do have many other nutritional benefits (enzymes in pineapple are great for digestion, for example) so there's no need to exclude them completely. At the end of the day, if you are quite overweight fruit is likely not the culprit, but for people who are already lean but wanting to reduce body fat further to expose more muscle definition, sugar consumption from all sources has to be taken into account. Fruit added to smoothies and shakes should be the whole fruit, chopped, but with edible skins left on.

Starchy carbohydrates

When talking about carbohydrates I am referring to 'starches' – grains, legumes, tubers (potatoes, parsnips etc.), plus bananas and, when eaten in large enough portions, squashes and other root vegetables. In the right amount (which is much less than we are used to consuming in our Western diet) they help satisfy hunger, cravings and boost energy, without negatively impacting fat loss. How much carbohydrate a person needs is down to the individual, so what we have recommended is an average portion for someone on a fat loss diet, then this can be adjusted according to how you are reacting by gauging hunger, cravings and energy levels throughout the day. Excluding carbohydrates completely is not recommended, as you will most likely struggle with one or all of the three main issues – hunger, food cravings or low energy – which will ultimately lead you to sabotage your efforts by binging on the wrong foods. Even vegetables contain carbohydrates and there is no need to restrict non-starchy vegetables. However, if you are feeling fine on the amount you are eating but are not losing fat, you could try reducing your starchy carb intake slightly at each meal.

WHAT TO EAT

Wholegrain or seed crackers or crispbreads are convenient and portable. Ezekiel bread is made of grains and beans, and is thought to be nearly as efficient as animal proteins, containing all 9 essential amino acids. It's a great alternative to bread, though still needs to be classed as a starch. Wholewheat bread and tortillas are also fine if you tolerate gluten. Legumes (beans, chickpeas, lentils) are high fibre, so a good starch choice. Grains such as barley, oats, couscous, and even quinoa – which is a 'complete protein' with all amino acids present – are all starches. Pasta and rice should preferably be wholegrain, or 'alternative' varieties, rather than white. Some 'vegetables' are actually starches too – white and sweet potatoes, Jerusalem artichokes, parsnips, broad beans and sweetcorn. The whiter the starch, the less you should have of it.

Tip: try eating more of your carbohydrate before and after exercise, and less on days you don't work out. They will help 'fuel' your workout and help replenish muscle glycogen, rather than be stored in fat cells if you don't burn them off through movement.

Condiments

Herbs and spices can be utilised to add flavour where salt, sugar and unhealthy trans fats have been cut out. In fact, some spices – namely cinnamon, ginger, chilli and cayenne – have been shown to aid metabolism and fat burning as well as reducing hunger, while cinnamon also helps balance blood sugar.

Vinegar (all types) is a surprisingly useful addition to anyone wanting to trim down. It slows down food transit time, making you feel full for longer, by triggering signals to your brain telling it you are full, and can even decrease insulin release after a carbohydrate-rich meal by more than 20%! All this points to reduced hunger, fewer cravings and less fat storage. Try adding a splash of balsamic vinegar before roasting vegetables, or as part, or instead of, salad dressing.

Salsa can add flavour and texture to foods providing it is a low sugar variety. Fresh salsa is mostly chopped vegetables (or fruit), water, herbs and spices, and vinegar.

Avoid lots of sugary sauces and condiments – barbeque sauce, cranberry sauce, etc. – unless using low sugar, or preferably sugar-free, versions. But finding ones sweetened with natural sweeteners as opposed to artificial ones will be hard, so you may want to make your own. Mustard and other unsweetened condiments are fine in moderation, as are small amounts of low-calorie sauces, like tomato ketchup.

While fat is vitally necessary to health, it is high in calories so can't be consumed in unlimited quantities. Mayonnaise and mayo based condiments when homemade, or very good quality bought ones, are OK in small quantities, the fat is not a problem, but they can add lots of calories very quickly. However mass produced shop bought ones can be highly processed with corn, canola and other, less desirable, omega-6 rich oils. Greek yoghurt with added herbs and spices, or natural flavourings such as mustard, makes a nice dip. Or alternatively drizzle a little oil-and-vinegar dressing over salads to add some nutritious unsaturated fat as well as flavour.

Sugar substitutes

Most of us crave sweet foods at times, but sugar (glucose, maltose, fructose, etc.), and even natural substances made up of different sugars, such as honey, maple syrup and agave nectar, are high calorie and very easy to overeat, send blood sugar and insulin levels soaring high, and fat storage can be the result of the easily eaten extra calories. Honey does contain many nutrients however, and most people can tolerate a little in treats; maple syrup and agave also contain nutrients, though not as much as honey; and agave nectar is, in fact, a long way from its plant origins and is very high in fructose, which is not good for your liver at all, but since we're aiming for low sugar consumption anyway you shouldn't need to use much if you do buy it. Low calorie artificial sweeteners are not recommended in abundance. They can stimulate hunger and cravings for sweet foods even further in some people, but know what works for you.

The best option is naturally derived low calorie sweeteners, which, thankfully, are becoming better known and more widely available these days, with most supermarkets stocking one form or another.

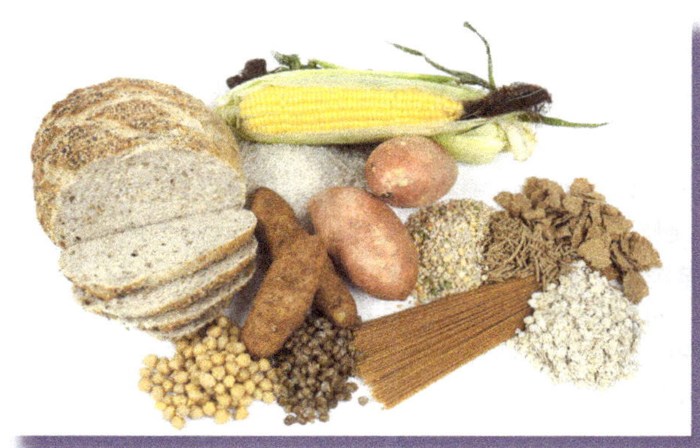

The following three natural sweeteners are naturally low calorie and are our favourite choices as you'll get your sweet hit without such big effects on insulin levels, cravings and hunger. Note that in some people even these cause them to crave sweet foods more and increases hunger, so, as always, know what works for you.

Stevia, a South American plant that is dried and ground to a sugar (or liquid extract) consistency, is becoming more popular because it does not affect fat storing hormones and may even have health benefits, such as being antiviral. Stevia is extremely sweet; a little goes a long way, although many commercial brands are bulked up.

Xylitol powder is a sugar alcohol that looks and tastes like sugar and can be a substitute for the same amount of sugar. Xylitol is actually made in the human body, as well as in birch tree bark and sweetcorn cobs. It slows digestion, making you feel full for longer, and protects against tooth decay.

Erythritol, which occurs naturally in fruit, is a sugar alcohol that is also a prebiotic, feeding the healthy bacteria in our gut and so benefiting digestion and nutrient absorption. Use 2 tsp. of erythritol in place of 1 tbsp. of sugar.

WHAT TO DRINK TO GET YOUR BODYBACK

Hydration is especially important when eating fewer carbs and salt, as these both retain water in your body. Drink at least 8 glasses of fluid a day, enough to keep your urine pale in colour.

Here is a list of The Fit Mum Formula approved drinks:

- water is ideal (preferably filtered but not essential); add a slice of lemon or lime to hot or cold water to make a change

- black tea (milk is fine but no sugar) has a small amount of caffeine for a pick-me-up, but also relaxing and rejuvenating properties; avoid in the evenings as it may disrupt sleep

- green tea is full of antioxidants as well as fat burning, metabolism supporting qualities that make it an excellent energy booster on a fatloss programme; avoid during the evenings due to the caffeine content

- herbal and fruit teas add flavour to water, and can have other benefits, ranging from energising, relaxing, immune boosting, appetite reducing or stimulating, diuretic, aiding digestion and more

- a mug of decent ground coffee (no more than three in a day), early on in the day, can help some people perform better in workouts and stay focused; it can also be an appetite suppressant, but for some people the opposite happens and appetite is stimulated, which is not so helpful; too much coffee can also increase stress hormones, and disrupt sleep

- cocoa powder, either added to coffee or a couple of tsp. topped up with hot water and a little stevia to taste, can stamp on cravings for sweet foods, as well as providing various minerals, and providing an energy lift

- alcohol is burnt like sugar, so will hinder fat loss; if you want to drink alcohol, have one measure (25ml spirits, 125ml wine, etc.) instead of your starch allowance for that meal; try to do this once or twice a week at most when your goal is to burn fat

- diet drinks and drinks with artificial sweeteners and additives are best avoided in excess, as these can stimulate hunger and cravings in some people, but as a calorie-free treat they're fine occasionally, if you like them

- fruit juice is not advised since it is concentrated fruit sugars but without the benefits of the fibre being present

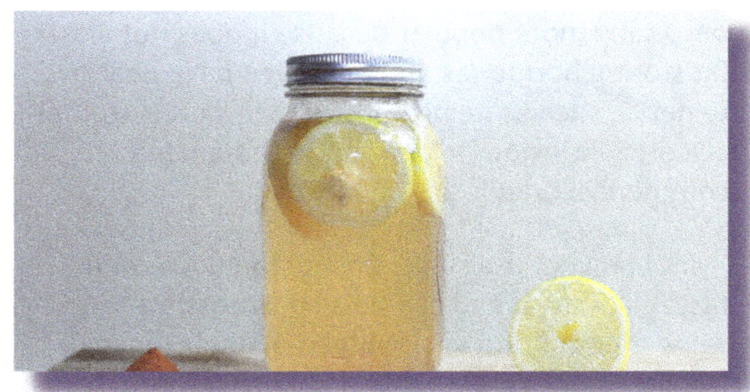

SHOPPING LIST

Here are a few items which are good to have in your fridge and cupboards, so that you always have something to hand to make a meal with in a hurry. The more variety you have the less bored you'll get and the more likely you are to really enjoy sticking with the programme. Obviously, how much/how many of these items you buy each week depends on how many people you have in your house to feed, and you wouldn't be expected to buy everything in one go as it's a long list, but you should always keep a stock of dried, tinned and store cupboard ingredients with long shelf lives. You can add other items to this list, and if you're in doubt as to whether it's a good choice feel free to contact me and ask.

VEGETABLES AND SALADS

Aubergine
Bean sprouts
Broccoli
Brussels sprouts
Carrots
Cauliflower
Celery
Courgette
Cucumber
Garlic
Green beans
Greens
Kale
Leeks
Lettuce
Mushrooms
Onions
Peas (frozen)
Peppers: red, yellow, orange or green
Pumpkin
Squash (all types)
Spinach (fresh and frozen)
Swiss chard
Tomatoes: chopped tinned, and fresh

FRUITS

Apples
Apricots
Bananas
Berries and cherries (fresh and frozen)
Grapefruit
Kiwi fruit
Lemons and limes
Melon
Oranges
Peaches
Pears
Plums
Rhubarb
Satsumas

PROTEIN

Beef jerky
Chicken: whole or breasts, raw or precooked
Eggs
Egg whites (carton)
Fish, oily: fresh or tinned tuna, salmon, sardines and mackerel
Fish, white
Lean beef: steak or mince
Meats, ready sliced sandwich meats (not re-formed)
Prawns, shellfish and seafood mix: fresh or frozen
Protein bars
Protein shake powder: whey or vegan alternative
Quorn or TVP products
Tofu (occasionally)
Turkey steaks or mince

STARCHY CARBOHYDRATES

Chickpeas and beans: tinned or dried
Crackers, bread and tortillas: wholegrain or high fibre, or grain free/seed/legume based.
Coconut flour
Lentils: tinned or dried
Oat bran
Oats
Parsnips
Quinoa: whole, flour
Rice: wholegrain
Sweetcorn, corn on the cob
White and sweet potatoes

DAIRY

Cheese: Parmesan, Cheddar, mozzarella, ricotta, cottage and cream cheese
Dried skimmed milk powder
Greek yoghurt
Milk: dairy or alternatives

FATS

Almonds, ground
Animal fats for cooking, e.g. goose fat
Avocados
Butter
Coconut oil
Desiccated coconut
Ghee
Nuts: whole, raw
Olive oil
Olives
Peanut butter (or any other nut butter)
Seeds
Vegetable oil spray

EXTRAS

Black peppercorns
Black tea

Cocoa powder

Granulated stevia

Green tea

Herbal teas (ginseng to energise, chamomile or lemon balm to relax)

Herbs: oregano, basil, rosemary, parsley, mint, coriander, etc.

Honey

Maple syrup (for baking if you choose to)

Mustard

Soy sauce

Spices: ginger, cinnamon, chilli or cayenne, curry powder, etc.

Stevia: granulated and liquid

Stock or stock cubes

Tomato paste

Tomato salsa

Vanilla Extract

Vinegars: balsamic, red and white wine

But some of those less common foods ...

... where on earth do I find them?

From coconut flour to stevia to ground chia seeds, these recipes use healthier alternatives to create delicious meals that are way more nutritious than using white flour and sugar. But while supermarkets are getting better at extending their healthy ranges they almost certainly won't have absolutely everything you need, so I created a solution – get everything you need that you can't find in your local shops at

www.thefitmumformulashop.com

I only stock food and supplements I personally approve of and use, so you don't have to worry that you might accidentally get some junk that's 'pretending to be healthy', big brands do a good enough job of that!

Some things you can find, in addition to the ingredients, linked from this book include:

- snacks, including bars and energy balls

- low carb gluten free pasta and virtually calorie free konjac noodles

- baking mixes

- high quality and tasty protein powders

- high quality vitamin and mineral supplements

- beef jerky and biltong

And loads more!

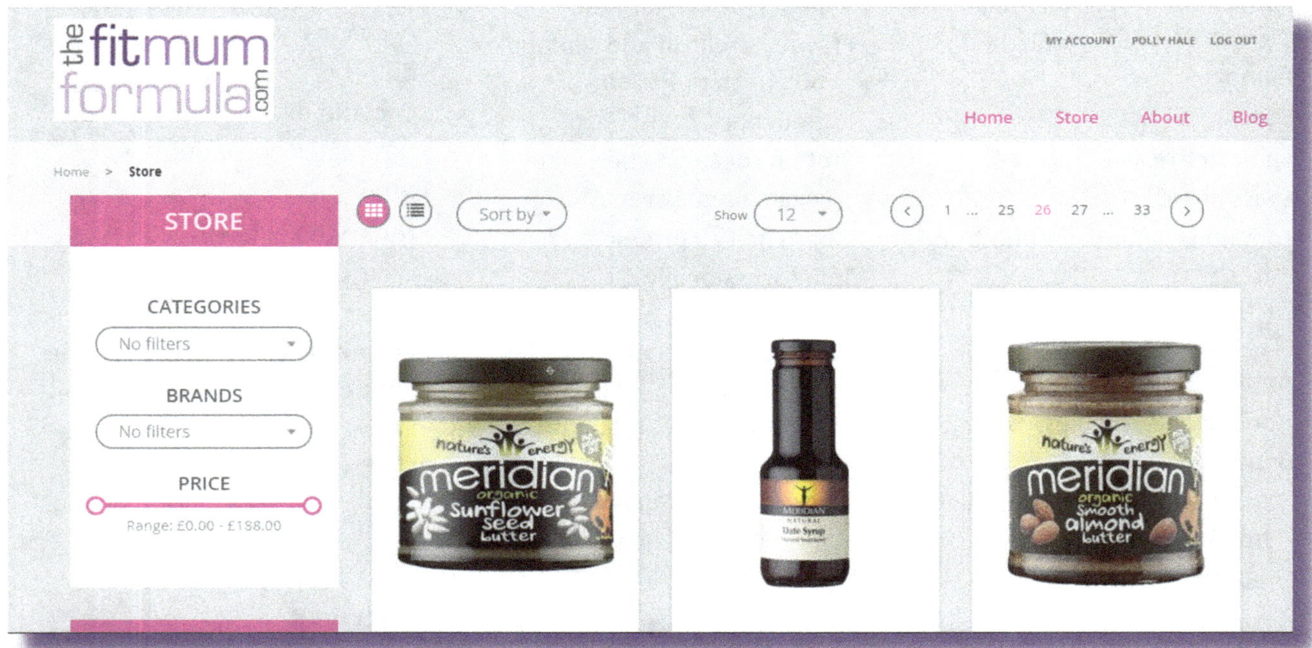

MINDSET

SWAP 'WHY' AND 'WHEN' FOR 'WHAT' AND 'HOW'

Call me stubborn, overambitious and idealistic, if you like. But my motto in life has always been that it's not about IF you can do something, only a matter of HOW. If you really want something, you will go to the ends of the earth to get it. If I held a gun to your head or told you that ws how to get the kidney donor your sick child badly needed, would you get results? Of course you would.

But before you tell me, "But I really can't get to the gym – I get home at 8pm and have to put my kids to bed", etc., etc., I'm not talking about trying to do things you can't do.

I'm talking about finding a way around this problem, finding a solution to the barriers, so that you can still achieve the same results.

If you loved exercise enough to have it high on your priority list you would find a way to fit it in, believe me you would. It's OK if you don't like exercise. You probably have negative memories and emotions attached to those memories.

Let me tell you about my experiences at boarding school again. I've always thrived in creative, agility sports – gymnastics, trampolining, ice skating, dancing. But running? Let's just say I figured out that if I just made it round the field during cross country I could sit in the woods for 20 minutes before running back, for a realistically timed finish. Turns out I had undiagnosed asthma all my life, which no doubt didn't help, which is triggered by damp air – dewy Cotswold fields and woodland come to mind. To this day running (by which I mean jogging, sprinting I love, sometimes) is a mental barrier for me, even though I have an inhaler on standby and the knowledge that I am, in fact, very fit. The answer? I don't run. I do other stuff.

On the other hand, some people will never like any sort of exercise. It's rare, but it happens. In this situation you have to evaluate what you really want.

Sometimes we have to do things we don't want to do to get the things we do want, or to avoid the things we don't want.

You go to work because you want to treat your family to a holiday. You brush your teeth because you don't want bad breath and rotten teeth. You do it for the end result, not just the process.

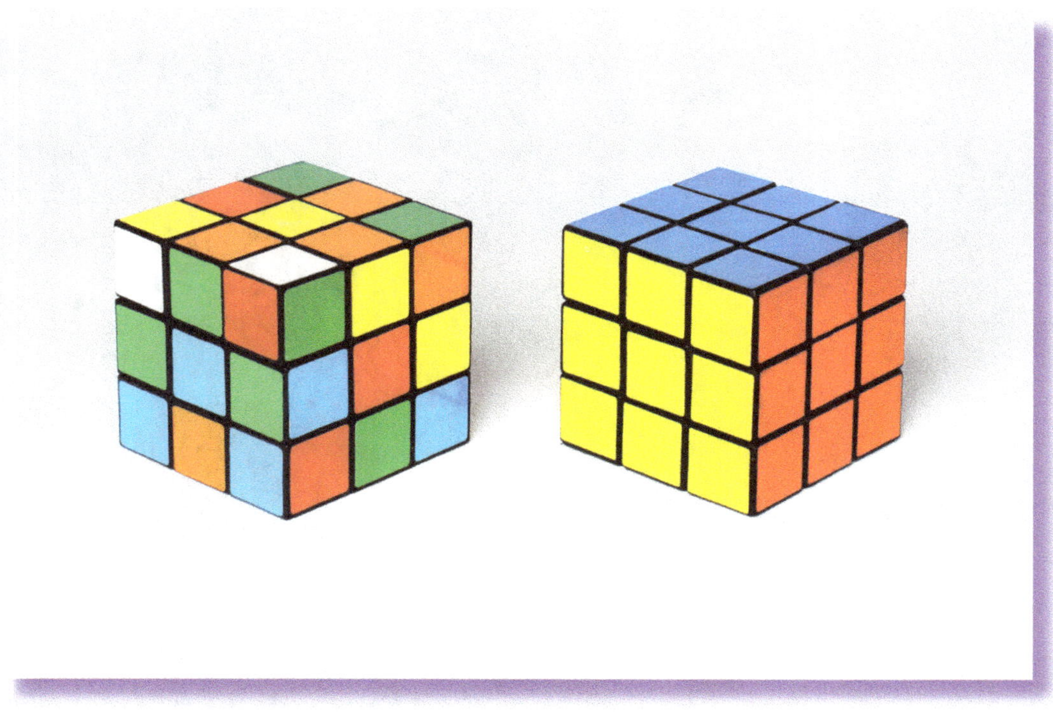

MY STORY – WHY YOUR MIND IS SO PRECIOUS

Why am I so passionate about being healthy in body and mind?

I nearly died of an eating disorder.

I've got to warn you, this is raw, and I don't mean uncooked, I mean emotionally raw. It might be a trigger for you. That's not a bad thing. It's an indication you have things you need to address.

I love food, especially food that makes you feel good. But I wasn't always like this, not by a long way. And it's important for me to be honest with you, and to be true to myself.

I'm hoping it will help other people just knowing they're not alone.

Why am I so passionate about health? Because I nearly died.

I hope you won't judge me. I hope instead you will see that I'm not perfect but I have learnt a LOT, and I hope I can pass this wisdom on to you.

What doesn't kill you makes you stronger, literally. The words 'strong not skinny' are my mantra for the way I eat and exercise, and in my 'coming out' video I show you why:

https://www.facebook.com/thefitmumformula/videos/1141103185941354/

For years I was devastatingly ill, both physically and mentally, with anorexia nervosa. Against all odds I recovered, and now nourish and strengthen my body to be the best it can be.

I now coach other women to get the body and the body confidence they want with online coaching.

Most women come to me wanting to lose weight not gain it. But it doesn't matter as it's all the same really, caring for your body and treating it well so that it becomes the body you deserve.

You only have one body, look after it.

In this next video I'll show you what can happen when you put your mind to overcoming something, however difficult.

Go here to watch my 'Strong Not Skinny' video:

https://www.facebook.com/thefitmumformula/videos/1196484663736539/

If these videos affect you in any way please share them so that we can raise awareness, and potentially inspire hope and courage in others who are struggling with their body.

THE FIT MUM FORMULA LIFESTYLE

In an ideal world, we would all like to be able to live to the following advice, but 'life' has a habit of getting in the way. Essentially, the important thing to take away from this is, if you know where you are going wrong, you will know what needs to change.

Sleep

Does sleep burn calories? You'd think not, given that you're lying down resting, even more than while watching TV. But you'd be wrong. Think about it: your heart pumps, your lungs expand, and the body does most of its repair work, be it to organs, skin, bone or muscle, while you are asleep, and all of these activities require calories.

But it goes further than that. Sleep also resets your hormones so that they are balanced and will play in your favour for overall health, not just fat loss. Lack of sleep causes the body to release more of the stress hormones adrenaline, noradrenaline and cortisol, which raise blood sugar, causing an insulin release to lower it again, and the cycle which leads to insulin resistance (diabetes) has begun, and you haven't even eaten anything yet!

Sleep also lowers the amount of the hormone ghrelin (hunger) in your bloodstream, while raising leptin, which makes you feel full, so you will be hungrier if you don't sleep enough.

Sleep also raises glucagon to break down fat stores, human growth hormone (HGH) and testosterone,

needed to build and repair muscle, which in turn is needed to burn calories and fat.

At least 8 hours sleep a night is required for optimum hormone balance, and is the simplest and most effective way to achieve the muscle-building, fat-burning, anti-ageing, mood-enhancing states that we so desire. Getting less than adequate sleep may seriously inhibit your ability to burn fat as fuel, and is the quickest path to muscle wastage, a saggy appearance, ageing skin, and generally poor health.

Problems getting good quality sleep?
Try these pointers:

- avoid too much caffeine; this is going to be different for each person – some people can sleep well after a coffee drunk well into the evening, while others have to avoid it completely, even in the morning

- make time to exercise; it will energise you in the short term, but come bedtime your body will more readily fall into a deep sleep

- don't go to bed too full; allow 2–3 hours between your main evening meal and bedtime, to allow your body to build, burn and repair, without having to worry about digesting food

- don't go to bed too hungry; a small protein based snack – such as milk, a small protein shake (1 scoop of powder with just milk or water), some cottage cheese or some raw nuts or seeds – before you go to bed can keep you satisfied through the night, and avoid you waking or stirring in the night due to hunger; it also delays catabolism while you sleep, which is where your body burns muscle to fuel itself

- if you don't get enough sleep then try to have a nap (20–30 minutes max is ideal or you risk eating into your evening bedtime), do 5 minutes of deep breathing, some meditation, yoga or tai chi, or go for a relaxing walk, all of which will help counteract the stress induced by lack of sleep

Light

It makes complete sense that as a human race we are designed to sleep when it is dark, and be awake when it is light. But with our modern lifestyles – work, children, hobbies and socialising – this is rarely the case these days. As much as it would be lovely to have the energy to be awake from 4am–11pm in summer, then sleep from 5pm-9am in winter (the latter offsets the former which makes it achievable), this just isn't realistic. However, we don't help matters much ourselves; we sit in front of the 'artificial light' – that is, the TV or computer – late into the evening, accompanied by bright overhead lighting. Lying in the next day doesn't help, since sleep/waking hormones are activated by light (or lack of light), if you sleep for 8 hours from midnight in the summer, only 4 or 5 of those are in complete darkness.

Studies have shown that stress hormones are at higher levels in people who go to sleep after midnight than those who nodded off before, even if their total sleep was the same amount of hours.

Aim to be asleep by 10, which probably means getting into bed a few minutes earlier to allow time to drop off, though don't worry if you're not sleeping; getting wound up will only make the problem worse!

Sunlight also prompts the body to make vitamin D (hence its nickname 'the sunshine vitamin'), which is not only important for bone health but is a great mood booster, and is why we all feel cheerier when the sun is out, and why some people suffer from seasonal affective disorder (SAD) during the winter months. Getting out into the sunlight is integral to our health, and even better if it's to go walking, as you'll be getting the tremendous benefits of that

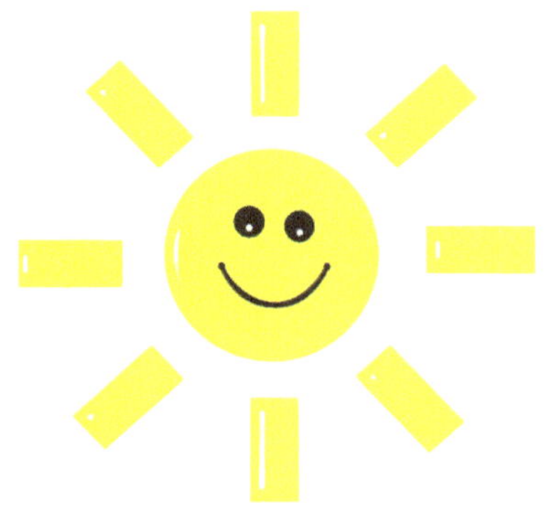

too. It doesn't have to be a 5am hike, the school run on foot will do! This is especially important during the darker, cloudier winter months, when vitamin D stores become depleted and a lowered mood could demotivate you into not looking after your health, which could lead to a vicious cycle. If you feel you're not getting enough light, even through proper sleep patterns and adequate time outside in daylight, try investing in a lightbox, which simulates sunlight and can help with mild to moderate SAD.

Stress

When we think of stress we think of having a bad day at work or the kids acting up, and while this is true, there are actually many things which act as stressors on the body, and cause it to release the stress hormones adrenaline, noradrenaline and cortisol. Not getting enough sleep, over exercising or exercising the wrong way, going too long without food, and too many stimulants (such as caffeine) all put the body under stress. This contributes to a decline in health, mood and energy and can give rise to symptoms such as increased heart rate and shallow breathing, increased perspiration, headaches and migraines, digestive problems, and emotional and psychological issues, as well as, of course, increasing hunger and cravings, and puts the body into a fat-storing and muscle-wasting mode, the opposite to what we are trying to achieve. The overall effects of stress should not be underestimated.

Stress has its place; the fight or flight response was crucial to the survival of prehistoric man, and we need it to react quickly if, say, a child runs into the road in front of us and we need to slam on the brakes. However, prehistoric stressors involved intense activity, like sprinting away from a predator, and this physical output offsets the stress response. You don't experience that physical exertion when slamming the brakes on the car, and this leads to an accumulation of stress hormones in the body, and all of the problems this brings about.

Stress affects your appetite and ability to digest food. Our body can only do so much at one time, so when we're under stress, such as after a break up, our adrenal glands pump out the stress hormones adrenaline and cortisol, which in turn elevate our blood sugar. Digesting food is not a priority when the body is trying to manage so many chemical changes in the body, so it turns down our appetite. It can go the other way though too; if these erratic blood sugar levels drop low, people experience cravings for sweet foods, typically in people who comfort eat. An interesting phenomenon is that there is a reason we turn to chocolate; the compounds in cocoa encourage the production of the neurotransmitters serotonin and dopamine, which make us feel happy and contented.

Now here is the interesting thing about cortisol. If cortisol is present when a) no physical exertion (intense exercise) takes place, b) insulin is also present (after consuming sugar or starch), or c) if glucagon is forcibly released (by going too long without eating), cortisol acts as a muscle-burning, fat-storing hormone. However, when in combination with HGH and testosterone, it becomes a muscle-building, fat-burning hormone. Three key things which increase both HGH and testosterone are: sleep, protein (and avoiding spikes in blood sugar levels), and intense exercise.

N.B. women will NOT bulk up like bodybuilders by doing resistance and weight training, we simply don't have the testosterone levels required to do this. Female bodybuilders work very had with very strict lifestyles to look like that, which is extremely difficult for most women to achieve.

How to minimise stress

- sleep enough, sleep deeply, and sleep at the right time (see above)

- walk as much as possible, leisurely not power walking, and among nature if possible, as the stress-busting effects are enhanced further when walking in the countryside, woodland, or even a local park

- do some intense exercise (The Fit Mum Formula workouts are ideal), which will turn cortisol into a fat-burning hormone as opposed to a fat-storing one

- minimise caffeine consumption if you think it is affecting you

- don't go longer than 3–4 hours without food; until your body is more able to reach for fat stores when you haven't eaten in a while, don't let yourself get too hungry as stress hormones will take over

- eat properly; highly nutritional, good quality foods fuel your body and brain and help you deal with stress more effectively; protein in combination with cortisol burns fat and builds muscle rather than storing fat

- let go of emotional and psychological stressors that you have little or no control over: road traffic, a boss who's in a bad mood, a broken washing machine for example.

- rather than getting wound up find solutions to stresses you have some influence over, like misbehaving children, an argument with a significant other, or a pile of paperwork to deal with

- do relaxing activities, such as yoga, tai chi, have a massage, read a book, etc.

- drink GABA-enhancing teas: chamomile, passiflora and lemon balm are all GABA (a relaxing neurotransmitter) enhancing

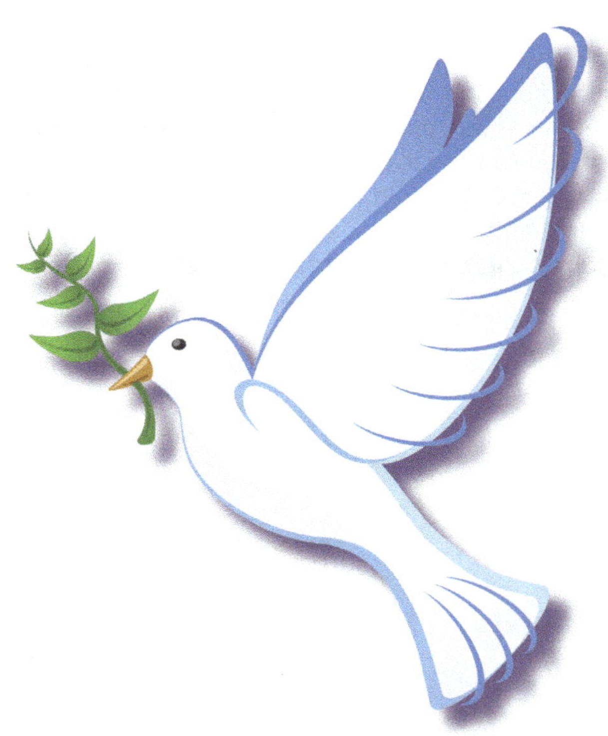

ON BEING A STRONG WOMAN

What comes to mind?

Female bodybuilders? Celebrities who have overcome huge challenges in the public eye? Olympic athletes? It will mean a different thing to different people, but hold that picture of your 'strong woman' in your mind.

Does that look like a woman who needs to stop eating all the pies and get off the sofa?

That's a woman who can take on the world.

To me, it's more than skin deep.

A Strong Woman is one who takes on challenges, faces their fears, is independent, and sure as hell has better things to worry about than what the number on the scale says. Because honestly, yes I help women lose weight if they need to (meaning lose fat, not muscle), but that's just the surface. The best result is someone who learns the skills to be strong both inside and out, and has the confidence to take on whatever the world throws at them.

Here's an odd phenomenon that I'm not sure how it works, but I've seen it enough times to know it does. There appears to be a correlation between strength of body and strength of mind. Think about it, when you're in bed with a stinking cold nothing seems possible. The opposite can also be made true. Maybe it's the self-efficacy of knowing you can achieve something. Maybe it's because after working out a while you're more confident about your body. Maybe it's exercise endorphins.

Honestly? I don't know. But I've seen enough women turn to exercise and it has radically, sometimes literally, saved their life. A strong and healthy body and a strong and healthy mind go hand in hand.

SET YOUR MIND FOR SUCCESSFUL GOAL-ACHIEVING

We talked about setting goals in the introduction. Did you do it? Did you write all the answers down and tick off everything on the checklist?

If not, stop reading, and go and do that now, before you go any further.

Because this book is not a novel for entertainment, I want you to take action.

If you have done your goal setting, plod on. We can take another look at making goals achievable.

Spring is another time of year when people make big changes. With Christmas over, the days getting longer and lighter, even the trees are starting afresh, you are re-evaluating what you want. Houses go on the market or are spring-cleaned, summer holidays are booked, and some people embark on the 'bikini diet' since the New Year's resolution didn't work out ;).

Lent is a traditional Christian festival when people give up things for 40 days. **The deprivation is a time for reflecting on what we do that's right or wrong, and exercising self-discipline.**

As with New Year's resolutions, anything that makes people look at themselves and their actions, and change them for the better has got to be a good thing.

The difference being that while at New Year statements to give up or start something new can be pretty generalised, Lent is a fixed amount of time; beginning on Ash Wednesday (the day after Shrove Tuesday) and ending on Easter Sunday.

It's been proven that **when we make resolutions with specific and fixed goals and terms, we are more likely to stick to them**, and that's why I think people are more successful at sticking to their 'giving up' over Lent than they are in the New Year, because they know it's not forever.

Are you seeing what I'm seeing?

If you were to say to yourself, "I will never eat chocolate cake ever again", how likely do you think you would be to honour that statement for the rest of your life?

How about "I will not eat chocolate cake for 40 days". Now THAT sounds doable. Just.

What about the rest of the year? How about:

"I will only eat cake on the weekend."

"I will only eat cake once a week."

or

"I will eat cake up to three times a week, but only have two mouthfuls each time."

Choose which you think will work for you, or think up your own, there are endless variations on this theme that can be applied to whatever your 'weakness' is. If it doesn't work, try a different one. By which I don't mean keep hopping between ideas and not sticking to them. Rather, the one you prefer best is the one you will likely stick to.

Sometimes abstaining completely, but temporarily, works best for people; if there's no choice, there's no internal debate, and the answer is simple, you don't eat it, and if that works for you then fine. Many people find that temporarily abstaining from something is all they needed to break the habit, and they find that after 40 days they didn't miss it so much after all, and continue their new habits for much longer.

Of course, at Easter those things called Easter Eggs have a habit of swaying even the most strong willed of us somewhat ... only once a year right?!

HABITS AND WHY I LOVE THEM

Habits are great. They are what people who are consistently fit and lean do. And the best bit? You don't even realise you're doing them! Because that's what a habit is, it's done unconsciously, automatically, without a second thought and is therefore completely effortless.

You've heard that 'diets' don't work, and the reason is lack of habit. Anything new, novel, quirky, strict, regimented or drastically different from what you are already doing is going to require a fair bit of effort on your part. You're out of your comfort zone, away from the familiar, and are certainly a long way from any of these new behaviours becoming habits.

The next problem with 'diets' is that they don't even need to become habits, because they are temporary. They assume – as stated in their marketing blub, and varying depending on the 'diet' in question – that either their 'diet' will give you the kick-start and motivation you need to continue, or that by following their 'diet' new habits will be formed.

But guess what? It doesn't work! Google it and you'll find 'studies' claiming it takes 21 days, or 30 days, or doing/not doing an action x amount of times for it to become a habit. Rubbish!

Sorry guys, but some habits, in some people, are for life, and you might have to watch your step over little habits for years before they genuinely become unconscious habits.

Your brush your teeth every morning (I hope). That's a habit. Or is it? I've been doing that for nearly 33 years at the time of writing (I don't actually know when my first teeth popped through, should ask Mother out of interest), yet every morning it is a conscious decision to walk into the bathroom and execute that action. I know that because on a weekend or in school holidays, when I don't have to jump out of bed and leave the house early, said teeth brushing might not happen until later, proving I did not automatically, in a sleep-walk-like state, brush my teeth without conscious thought.

Here's the good news. Habits are not all or nothing, black or white. Behaviours can be more or less consciously done, depending on where they are on the habit scale.

And the longer you persist with certain behaviours the more they move up the habit scale, so they are done with less and less thought, and are more and more automatic, and you are less likely to forget, trip, stumble and behave in the 'old way'.

Also, you are in a much better place (very likely in fact) to be able to have the odd 'deviance', be that a chocolate biscuit, ignoring your workout routine for a week on holiday, or (shock!) not bothering to brush your teeth one night, and yet still go back to your 'good' habits straightaway after, without one deviance making you completely scrap well-intended plans .

So what does this mean for people wanting to eat better/exercise more/be healthier in general?

Keep going. Just keep doing it. If you don't do it one day, do it the next. Who said your journey or path has to be as straight and smooth as a Roman road? OK, so the Roman's might have got there quicker, but life is a journey. It's the journey that counts not just the destination, and sometimes the mistakes you make along the way, the twists and turns, backward steps as well as forward and sideways ones, provide some wonderful scenery and opportunities for learning. Maybe these learning opportunities even put you in a better place eventually anyway. Perhaps you'll stay at your new, healthier destination for life, whereas maybe the Romans got there in double time but came home just as fast, as they'd not learnt anything on their journey.

I digress. Sort of.

Two steps forward, one step back. Five steps forward, two steps back. You get there in the end, and every inch, foot, mile you achieve makes the habits move up that habit-ometer (great word huh?!) and they become slightly more subconscious thoughts, decisions and actions. My, then, 16-month-old was so reluctant to walk at first, even though we knew she could. She would only do it if encouraged and praised by everyone in the room. She just wouldn't 'get started' by herself. Then she did start, did a bit more, fell down, got up, tried again, tripped again, got up ... now she walks everywhere without a second thought, and only reverts back to wanting to be carried when very tired or ill. At age 4 walking is now a genuine habit for her, but only because she kept going, picking herself up after every trip and going again.

Don't feel guilty, what a waste of energy. Use every trip as a learning experience, pick yourself up and go again, until you find you're tripping less and less, even without more thought being put in than previously. What you are witnessing there, when you are tripping less, is at last, the slow but steady formation of a habit.

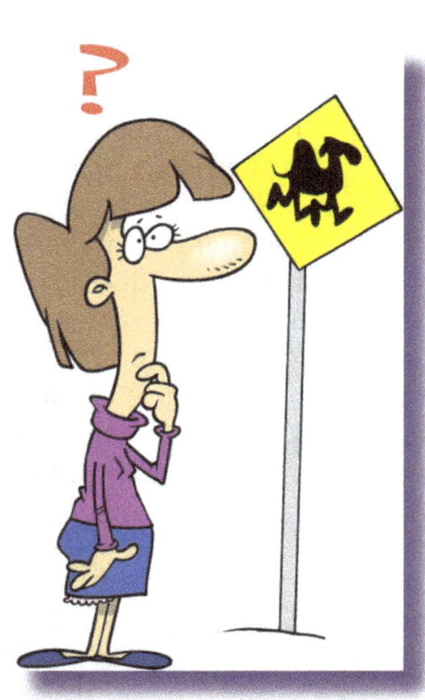

THE SUBCONSCIOUS MIND

You are one person, but you have many levels, and understanding these is necessary to understanding how you can exert control over your life, rather than life happening 'to' you.

It's a sequence of events. Let's start with your conscious mind. This is the rational, evaluative, thinking mind that understands and knows. It knows you should probably not eat a third slice of chocolate cake. It knows that swapping a bottle of wine for a glass would be a great improvement.

Yet here's the thing about the conscious mind; it knows, but it does not do

This is why many very smart people cannot get ahead in life. Their conscious mind is in peak condition, yet it's not the conscious mind that determines their actions.

Underneath the conscious mind is the subconscious. The subconscious stores memories and emotions. It does not rationalise or use logic. It accepts any idea or concept fed to it from the conscious mind. It is the dutiful worker to the conscious boss. Stories, ideas, words are all given to the subconscious mind from a very young age, as soon as you are born in fact. It does not question or reject thoughts, it simply accepts them and passes the message on to the body, which then acts.

The subconscious mind instructs the body to act, most of what you do on a daily basis is subconscious

So why do you continue to do things that are sabotaging your mental or physical health even though your rational, conscious mind knows otherwise? Because it wasn't your conscious mind that drove the decision, it was your subconscious.

Let's take an example. On your journey to losing weight in the past you have struggled with eating at restaurants. You consciously want to and know it would be helpful to choose a healthier dish. But you get overwhelmed by the menu, and persuaded by your meal guests to 'live a little', but rather than just choose something nice, enjoy it until you're full, and leave it at that, it turns into an all-out loss of control that includes an entire bread basket, bottle of wine, a side of cheesy potato gratin and a sticky toffee pudding. There is no middle ground or compromise when you eat at a restaurant, never has been.

Because this is how history has played out, this is the story you tell yourself. Even though you would like it to be different, this is what you believe is likely to happen. Your 'belief' is in your subconscious, where it will directly tell your body to act on that belief without question. Even when your conscious mind wants something else, remember that's not who makes things happen, it's your subconscious that does.

The conscious mind impresses thoughts into the subconscious. The subconscious then instructs the actions by the body. So how do we get out of this?

We change the thoughts that are being impressed upon the subconscious

The first time you got in a car to learn to drive you could barely start the thing. Next time you started OK, but when you tried to move forward you jumped and stalled. Then you crawled at a snail's pace. Soon enough you could travel smoothly along 20mph roads, even turning corners and stopping at traffic occasionally, without drama. Today, you don't even have to think about it, most of the act of driving has become subconscious (keeping an eye on the road and anticipating other cars/kids in the road is still conscious, and always should be). Do something enough times, and with enough intent and desire for the outcome (getting your driver's licence), and the conscious can impress new thoughts into the subconscious.

But there's a problem. Your subconscious mind is very much stuck in its ways, because it feels comfortable there. To change is to get out of the comfort zone, which feels weird, awkward, scary, terrifying even. If that sounds far-fetched, it's probably an indication that you've never, or very rarely, attempted to get out of your comfort zone by challenging your subconscious thoughts. It is not an easy thing to do, if done right.

Every time your subconscious is challenged, the fear arises and the easiest thing to do is to scrap the idea and continue to believe the thoughts and feelings that have kept you feeling safe, even if they're not keeping you happy, or as happy as you could be.

Impressing new thoughts from your conscious on to your subconscious is not as easy as repeating mantras every day. They're just words, and saying them does not automatically impress them into your subconscious, though it's a start.

How to change your subconscious

1. Pick one belief, anything negative you have about yourself. Perhaps that you never follow anything through to the end, or that you have no willpower.

2. Create a sentence that's the opposite of that, in the present tense, as if it is true today, rather than it will be in future, such as, "I complete all tasks and plans thoroughly to the end" or "I am a very strong-willed person".

3. Get a piece of paper and write it down 10 times. Cut these up and place them around, where you will be able to see it, a lot. In your purse, on your bedside table, on your desk, in your diary, on your fridge door, wherever you think you will see it.

4. Read it out loud every day. Believe it and feel it (this will be hard at first, just keep persevering).

5. Look for evidence that it is true. Did you complete a task at work today? Did you make yourself get up when your alarm went off, even though you'd have rather stayed in bed?

6. Repeat, repeat, repeat, until your actions start to change with less conscious effort on your part. This is an indication that the message is becoming more subconscious.

THE CAVEAT

This is not excuse to stop making conscious decisions. Healthy meals won't make themselves. Your workout won't happen if you don't actually get into your clothes and start doing something, or take yourself to the gym, or go for that walk. But these things are a big effort at first. They are conscious choices. The aim is to stamp them into your subconscious so that you do them without question, without thinking. They have become a part of your life. You'll wake up 30 minutes early on a Tuesday and make a coffee, drink it while you get into your sports bra and shorts, turn the computer/DVD player on, and do that workout before breakfast. Why? Because that's just what you do on a Tuesday, no questions asked. You don't even stop to think about the 'ifs' and 'whys' anymore. You just do it, because the belief that this is who you are and what you do is now in your subconscious, therefore the action has become automatic. And that is when healthy living becomes, honestly? Pretty easy!

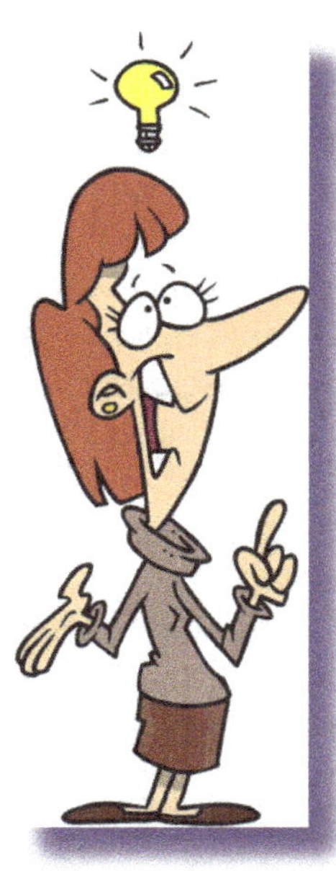

10 LESSONS LEARNT FROM A WORLD-FAMOUS DOCTOR

It's not often you get to spend the day with a world famous naturopathic doctor, but when you do, you sure as hell make sure you come away knowing more than when you woke up that day.

Dr Terry Wahls is infamous in the world of natural medicine, known best for using the Paleo diet to manage autoimmune conditions such as multiple sclerosis (which Wahls herself suffered from). But her approach is also used to help other conditions, such as diabetes, fertility, digestive issues and skin conditions, or simply just for people wanting to have more energy and feel better in themselves generally. I would recommend seeing a naturopathic doctor with experience in successfully using a dietary approach to illness, at least alongside your GP, since GPs don't get the training required to understand how powerful a medicine food can really be.

The Paleo diet involves eating meat, fish, eggs, vegetables, fruit, nuts and seeds. No grains, dairy, legumes or processed food are allowed. Some people do a more relaxed approach, eating organic dairy and beans too.

I was at the conference helping out for the day as, being a health professional myself, I would be able to help visitors with any questions they might have. It would have been easy to focus on the food advice, but that's quite simple really. In fact, I pretty much summed it up in the paragraphs you just read, and in the previous chapter on food.

So rather than tell you to eat healthy food (you know that), I thought I'd tell you the things that really struck me as significant, in ways we often forget to consider.

Here are some thought-provoking ideas I took away from the day. You might want to revisit this section every so often, as some of them take a bit of pondering over and time to digest, if you'll excuse the pun.

1. You have immense control over everything you do: where you live, what you eat, your physical activity, who you spend time with, even your thoughts.

2. Learnt helplessness is the belief that you do NOT have this control. Thankfully this negative belief can be unlearnt.

3. Nothing happens in isolation. Mental health, gut health, immunity, metabolism, stress, fertility … it's all interrelated.

4. You may have 'stuff' that holds you back – illness, lack of time, money, etc. – you also have many things in your life that can push you forward. Focus on those.

5. Consider how you can help others via helping yourself. If you are happier and healthier, you will be a better mother, a better partner, daughter and friend. You'll probably even start making your family healthier food for starters. You will also be an inspiration to others wanting or needing to improve their health. Pay it forward.

6. To be a hero is to separate yourself from the 'normal' crowd and take your own path, because the 'norm' is not serving you (or them). Lead the way.

7. Do not underestimate the power of relationships. Surround yourself with people who support and encourage you to improve your health, rather than ones who try to steer you off track.

8. Stress is not bad. Too much bad stress is bad. Stress is a much bigger contributor to poor health than you likely think.

9. Health choices either take you closer to, or further away from, your goals. Rarely are they neutral.

10. Pretty much every health condition, from the mildly annoying to the serious, can be at least helped, if not cured, through lifestyle choices alone.

What do you think?

Any in particular that resonate?

82 MOTIVATIONAL DAILY QUOTES

In my free Facebook Group and in my private member's group, I have a weekly spot for all things mindset and motivation, which, as you've read in this chapter, is as important as all the exercise and nutrition help I provide, along with accountability and support.

I've rounded up the best from the last six months here. They work best if you take some time to ponder and let them sink in, and take action on what you have learnt. You might like to read a couple a day, instead of all at once at the risk of forgetting them.

And if any particularly stand out or resonate with you? Feel free to highlight them, or write them down on sticky notes and stick them up where you will be reminded.

1. 20 steps to stay motivated

1. Chart your progress; measure results and check you're on track.

2. Hold yourself back; don't use up all your energy and motivation in the first week, go steady and slow.

3. Join an online (or off-line) group to help keep you focused and motivated – you can do that on https://www.facebook.com/groups/weightlossandfitnessformums/! But my BodyBack members get their own exclusive group too.

4. Post a picture of your goal someplace visible – a picture of you looking well and happy, maybe on your fridge?

5. Get a workout partner or goal buddy – or join an online club (see above).

6. Just get started. It all gets easier from there.

7. Make it a pleasure. Enjoy tasty healthy food, not boring healthy food!

8. Give it time, be patient. Consistency will bring results in time.

9. Break it into smaller, mini goals. Start with today.

10. Reward yourself. Often. Just not with food!

11. Find inspiration, on a daily basis. Follow people who are where you want to be.

12. Get a coach or take a class. We all need a little guidance now and again.

13. Have powerful reasons. Write them down. It makes them more concrete.

14. Become aware of your urges to quit, and be prepared for them. Have a plan in place for emergencies!

15. Make it a rule never to skip two days in a row. Keep the good habits going.

16. Visualize your goal clearly, on a daily basis, for at least 5–10 minutes. This isn't woo woo magic, it's just making sure your goals and plans are clear in your mind.

17. Keep a daily journal of your goal. Sssess how you're feeling, note any struggles, offload.

18. Create a friendly, mutually-supportive competition. Join up with others (see points 3 and 5).

19. Make a big public commitment. Be fully committed. Tell your friends and family, or post it on social media.

20. Always think positive. Negativity is contagious, don't spread it.

Which one is your fave?

I like no. 15. I'm a creature of routine and habit – good habits for the most part!

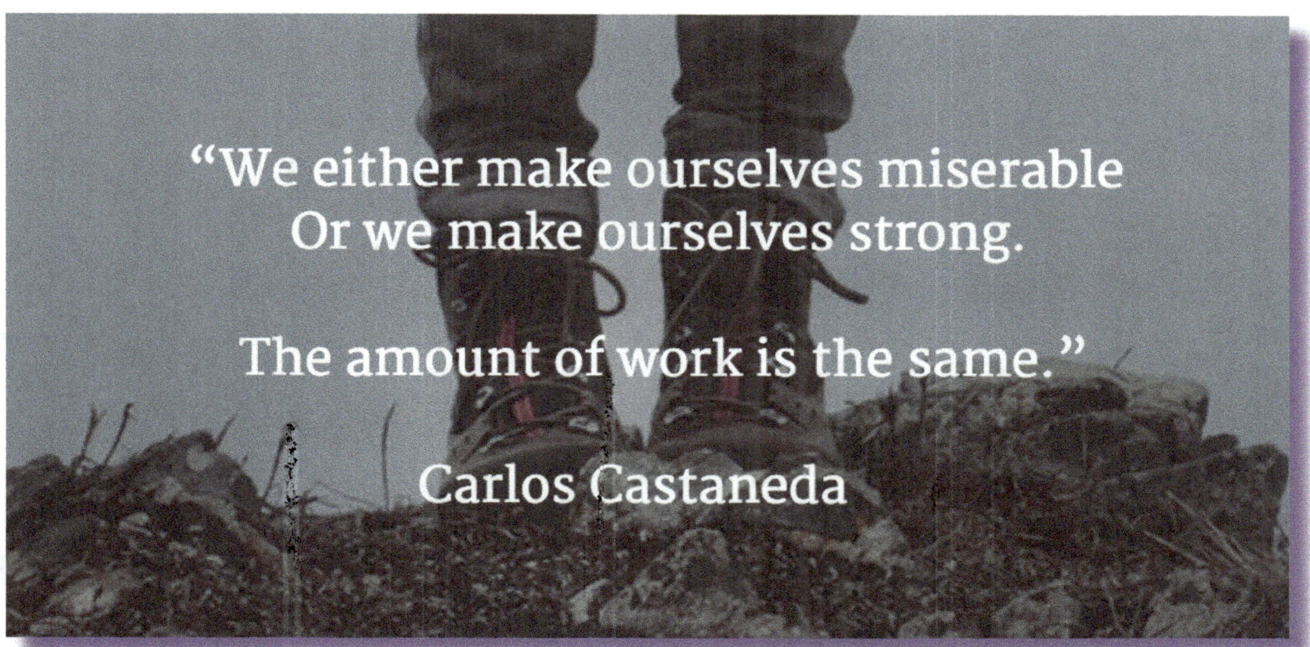

One of the biggest barriers to achieving your health and fitness goals is lack of time and energy. But have you considered that some of the time and energy you do have is being spent on the wrong things, things that halt or reverse progress?

Of course there's a place for eating cake and slobbing in front of the TV. But if you swapped just one piece of cake a week for an apple, and just one half hour show for a few home body weight exercises, then you're one step closer to your goals with no more time and effort spent.

Have a think? Is there a swap you can make in your week that makes you progress?

Are you preparing your environment to make it easier to stick to your plan or goals?

If you want to eat healthily, does your shopping trolley reflect this?

If you want to do a workout, have you put it in your diary and made sure your exercise clothes are ready to hand?

If you want to go to bed earlier, have you got organised to make this happen?

I'm not sure there are many people who can be successful all the time without at least a little forward thinking. Preparation will make success way more likely!

What do you do to make sure you follow through with your intentions?

We sometimes get an Ocado vegetable and fruit box; they're generous for the cost and we never run out of fresh fruit or veg.

I also like to lay out all my workout things, including water to drink and preworkout supplement (not essential but optional), the night before. Early morning stress doesn't need to be added to when I know the school run is imminent!

> "If you keep telling the same sad, small story,
>
> you'll keep living the same small sad life."
>
> Lee Iacocca

Who knows someone who is always complaining about their life/weight/circumstances, yet never does anything about it?

You probably know a few. Since you're taken the initiative to read this book you're not really in that category; that's at least one step you've taken toward change. But you can read all the posts, blogs and articles, watch the videos, listen to podcasts and talk to experts to get advice. Only that's not what's going to move you forward, there's only one thing that does that ...

ACTION

Most people have more than enough information. We have information overload, the result being INACTION through confusion.

Pick something – a decision to have a side salad with every meal, only to have take-away once a week, a 20 minute walk during your lunchbreak – whatever. Just choose one thing and do it.

When that becomes a daily habit that doesn't require so much effort?

THEN look for the next thing to add in.

Less talking, more doing.

"EXERCISE IS A CELEBRATION OF WHAT YOUR BODY CAN DO,

NOT A PUNISHMENT FOR WHAT YOU ATE."

For those of you who are trying to burn 'x-hundred' extra calories a day to speed up weight loss (many people have messaged me about this recently), this one is for you.

Of course calories matter, and of course you need to burn more (or eat fewer) to lose weight. But exercise doesn't burn as much as the DVD's/machines/trackers would have you believe compared to not exercising. If you burnt off 100 calories, chances are you would have burnt at least 70 just doing the supermarket shop or whatever anyway (made up numbers, just as an example).

Also, what happens if weight loss doesn't happen, or as fast as you'd like? Does that mean 'exercise doesn't work' or that you're wasting your time?

Exercise should be a joy (or at least the way you feel when you're fit is!) not a punishment. Cross country at school, THAT was punishment for me.

My The Fit Mum Formula workouts in my PJ's at 6am in my living room? Therapy; my sanity, ME time, where I can push out all the stresses, and the world feels like a better place. The fact that I look not too bad in a strappy top is pure coincidence. A bonus.

Talk to any supermodel and they're not happy all the time. But see a photo of Jessica Ennis with a Gold medal round her neck, that's pride and happiness in all its glory. And she looks pretty damn good too!

"Do not think that what is hard for you to master is humanly impossible; but if a thing is humanly possible, consider it to be within your reach."

– Marcus Aurelius

Apart from offering you a picture of a sexy man (always called for), have you ever given up hope on something because you thought it was too difficult to achieve?

Let's consider the difference between difficult, and impossible.

The first, by definition, is possible. Therefore it becomes not a case of IF, but HOW. Everything becomes possible when you know HOW.

Think you'll never be a certain size clothes, or will never be able to run further than the end of your street?

Can you turn these IF's into HOW's?

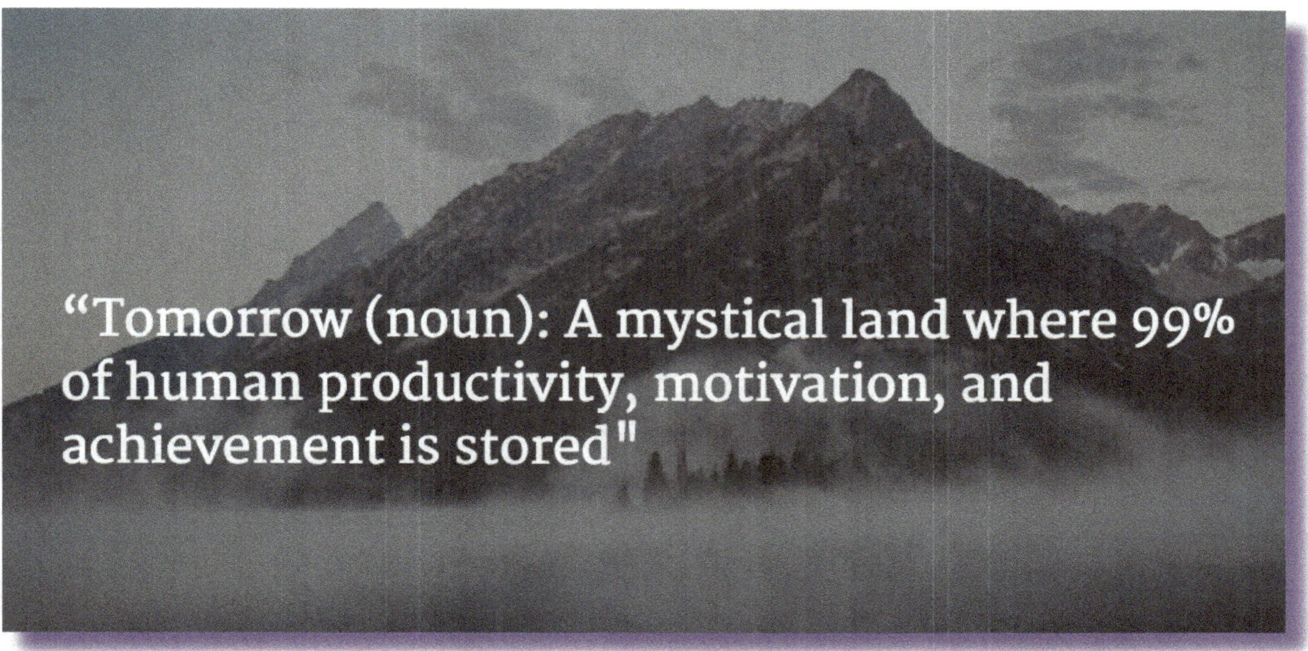

Who's guilty of this?

So, Monday has already started and you're planning on buying that new healthy cookbook during your lunch break, looking through it this evening, shopping for ingredients tomorrow, and making your first healthy meal tomorrow evening.

Well, what's wrong with today? You don't have to make some Instagram-worthy spectacular restaurant style dish to be healthy.

Keep it simple, make the most of what you've got, but most importantly, start NOW.

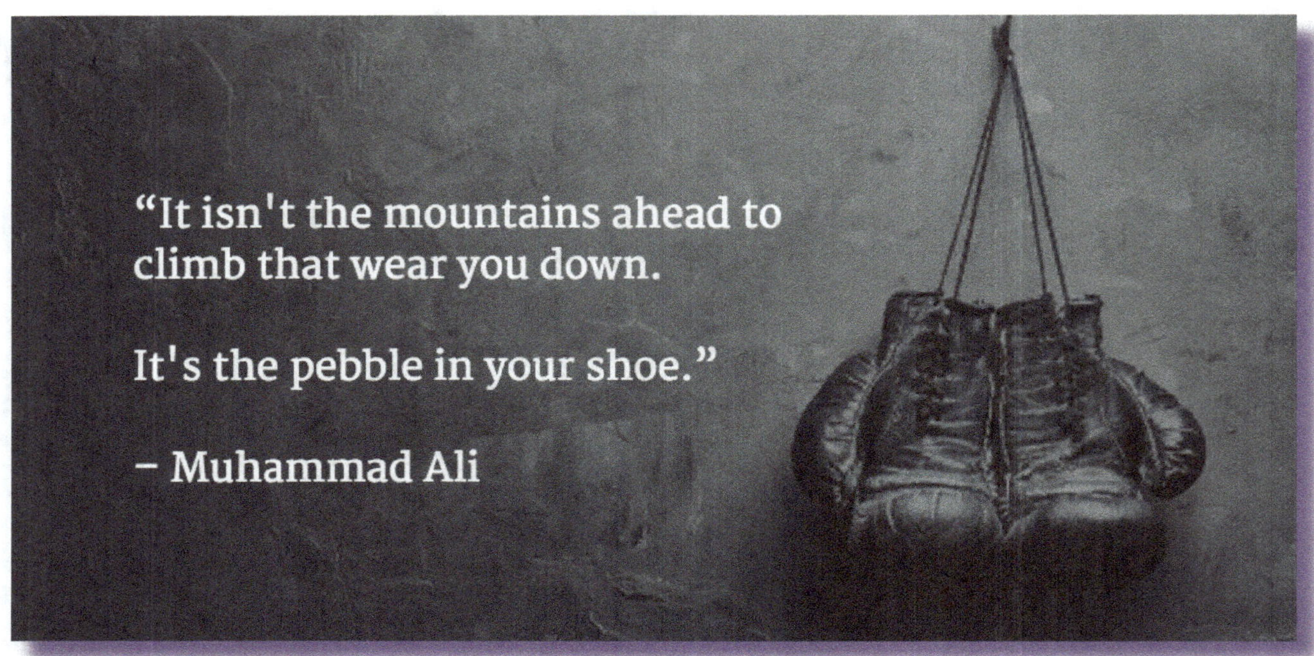

Is it the bigger goal seeming insurmountable that's preventing you from doing what you need to do?

I'd guess not, in fact, visualising your slimmer/fitter/more energetic self is highly motivating.

No, it's the little things in everyday life that get in the way: the child who is ill; the toys all over the floor to pick up; the washing spilling over the laundry basket that needs to be dealt with; the 'can't face the Supermarket with kids in tow' so eating frozen pizza instead (because it was there, and it's easy, and they won't complain for once)

The little daily things that stand between you now and where you want to be. But that actually makes them easier to deal with, because now the 'problems' can be broken down into small manageable tasks to overcome.

- keep frozen salmon and peas and sweet potato wedges in the freezer

- pay the kids pocket money for sorting the washing into colours (this might take some tweaking afterwards, but it'll keep them busy)

- dump all the toys into a plastic storage tub just to get them out of the way and deal with them AFTER your workout

- keep your workout clothes clean and easy to find

- and – my favourite – give them an iPad and tell them to be quiet for 30 minutes because Mummy needs some me-time (home workout) with a promise to do x/y/z afterwards, but only IF they let you have 30 minutes to yourself. Use the phrase "Yes/Maybe (depending on how ridiculous the request), but we'll discuss it when I've finished my workout, IF you can play by yourselves for the next half an hour, deal?"

Honestly, your kids will get used to you taking time for yourself, and after a while they might even stop interrupting you (as much, anyway)!

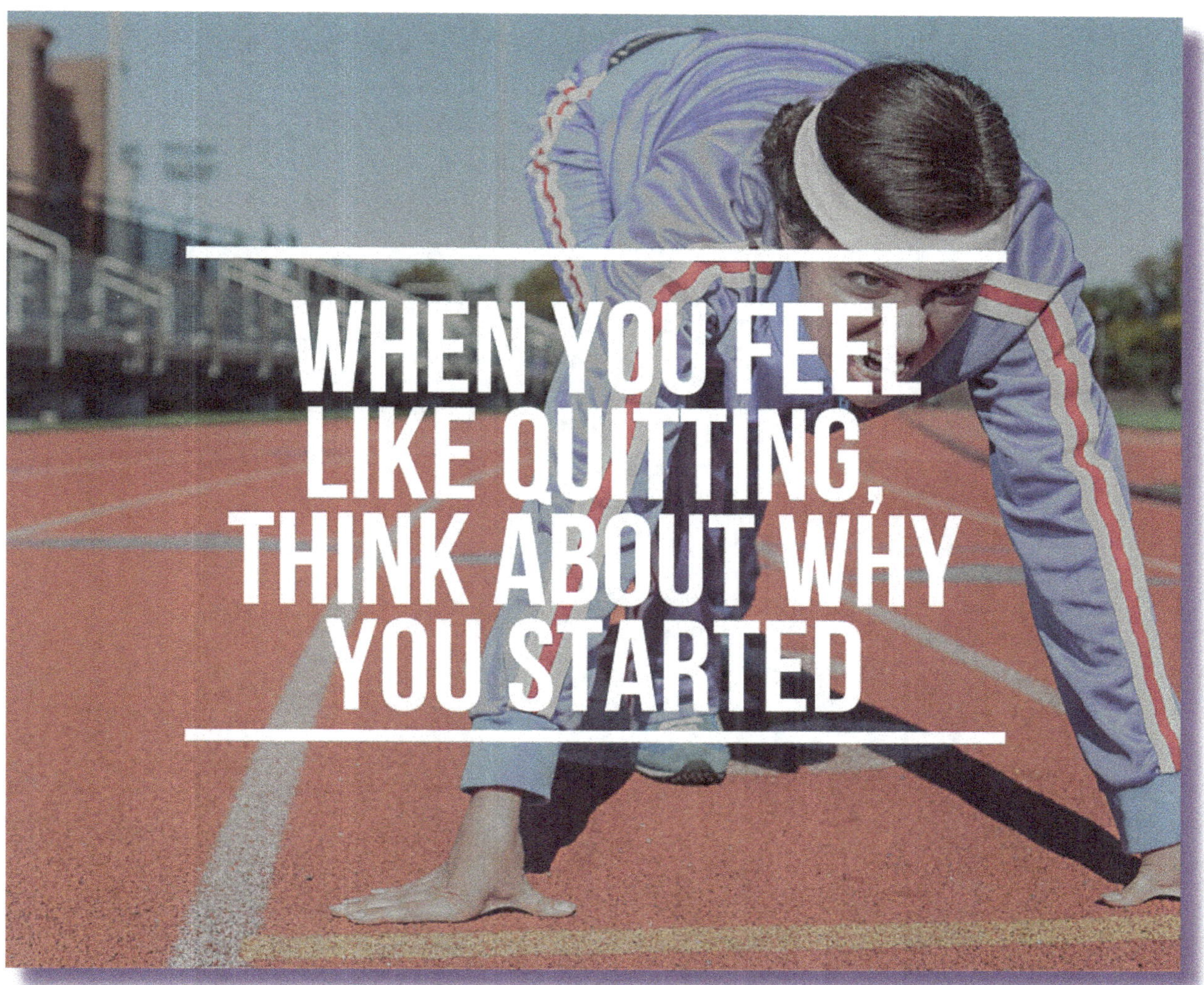

Monday is when people like to 'start the diet', how odd is that? It's not like your body understands the days of the week.

The reason likely is, our brains like order. They like structure and routine. They compartmentalise things to make them easier to recall – it's less strain on your brain so you have more mental energy left to devote to other things.

According to some studies five weeks is the duration most people stick on a diet before giving up.

I have two thoughts here. The first relates to the meme here, your goal (to fit back into your jeans, to feel confident at a wedding, have more energy to keep up with your kids, etc.) can easily get forgotten when you're stressed out (dieting), so keep photos (of a former slimmer self), objects (a smaller dress you've bought to wear to the wedding), and concrete goals (a date to go to the trampoline park, where you'll have the energy to join in!) within sight. It will remind you why you started in the first place.

The second thought is, if your 'diet' really is that difficult and horrible you want to quit, you're doing it wrong. Honestly, eating fewer calories doesn't have to mean you skip every treat that you pass, going hungry, feeling grumpy (hangry?!) and miserable.

Eating well should make you feel good. If it's not, it's time for a rethink of your strategies.

If you don't know how to eat well while still feeling good you're in good company. It's why most 'diets fail', then look back over the Food chapter, or feel free to get in touch with me for a chat.

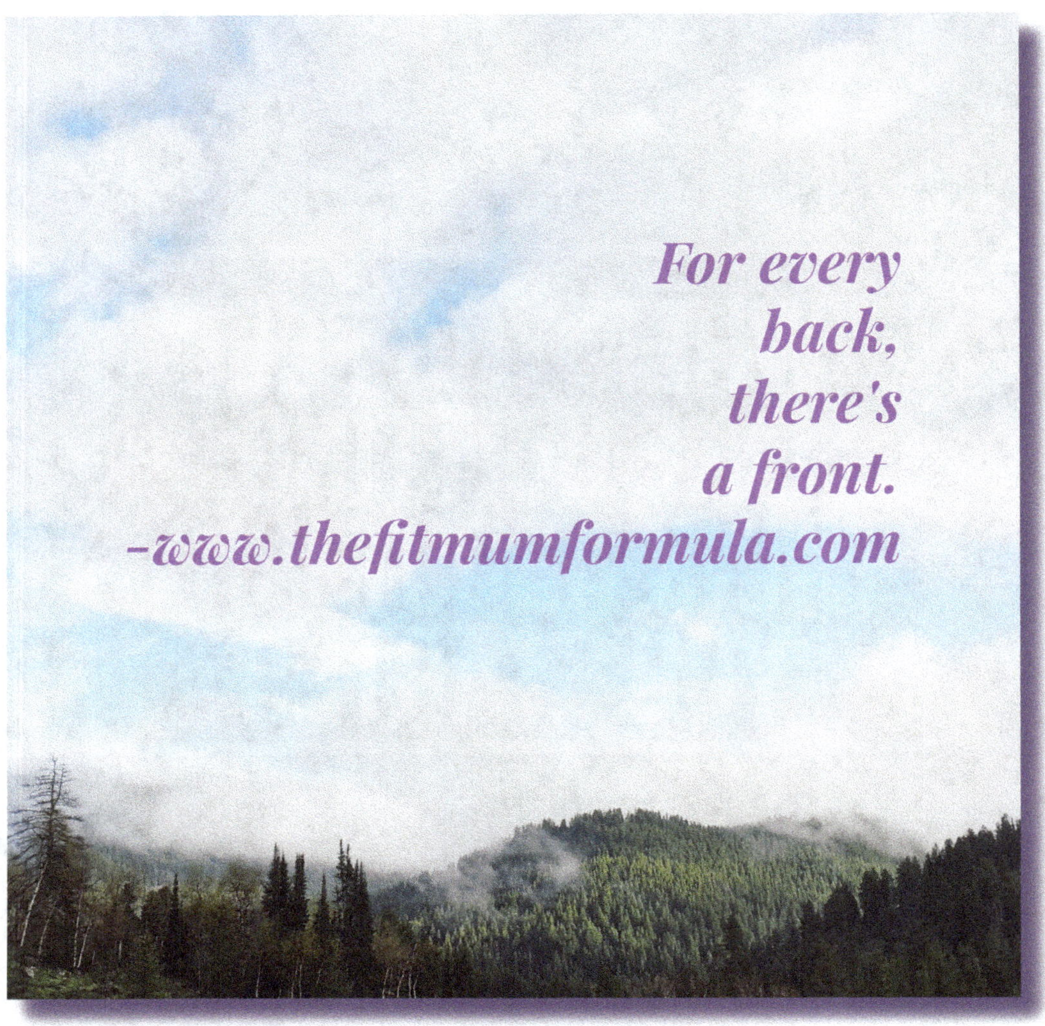

We all have a past, even just yesterday is in the past.

That doesn't matter.

It's now and tomorrow that counts.

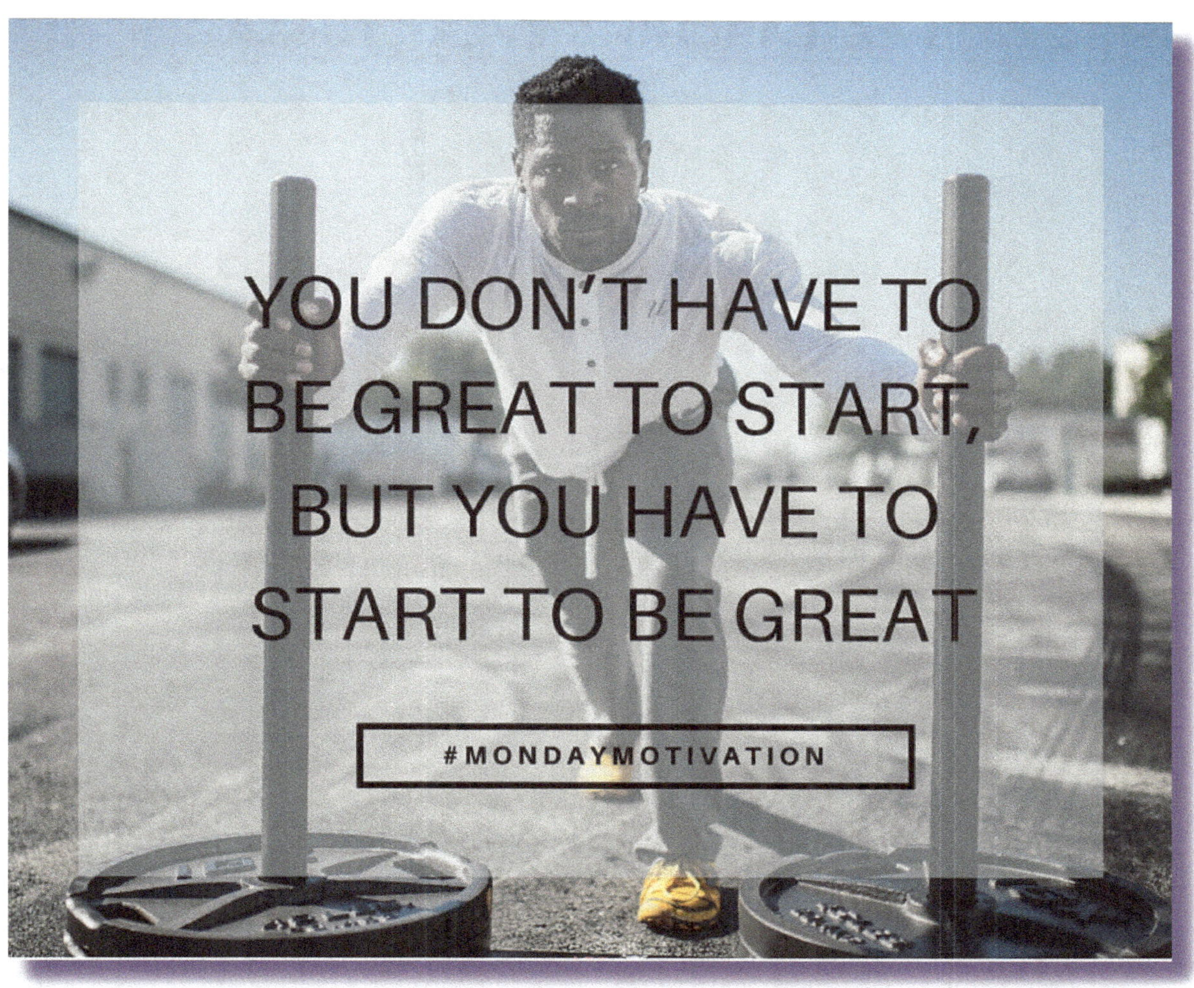

Have you ever felt too embarrassed to exercise in public because you're 'too out of shape'?

Or perhaps you wanted to read up a bit on healthy eating before deciding which sort of diet to follow?

These thoughts are procrastination and are holding you back. It doesn't matter where you start, just start somewhere.

Everyone who has ever succeeded at anything was a beginner once. Me included, obviously. I even owned one of those stupid 'electrocute your tummy' ab contraptions once, because I had no idea what I was doing!

Just start.

"TRYING BEATS RESEARCHING EVERY TIME."

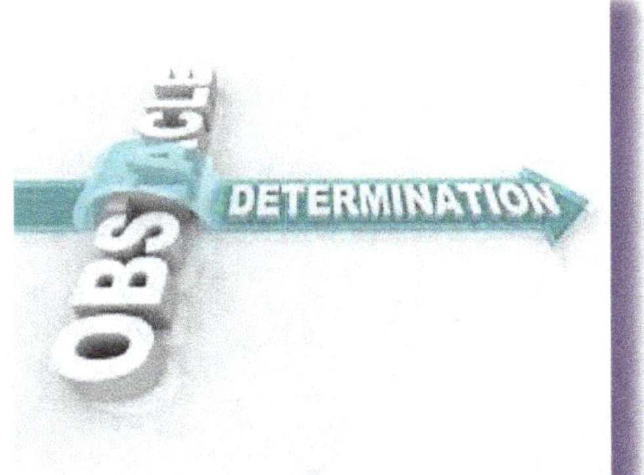

Research, then commit to something to reap the benefits of experience. Stop trying to gather secondhand diet information from other people. They don't know what works best for you, and you won't either without experience.

"YOU CAN DO ANYTHING, WITH THE RIGHT REASONS."

Warning, shocking analogy ...

Imagine your children are locked in a building. The building is on fire. And your kids are trapped.

You are told the only way to free them is if you can stick to your healthy eating plan (whatever that is), do a set amount of specific exercise and lose X amount of weight.

Could you do it? Of course you could. Such is the power of the mind and motivation.

Nothing changed in your circumstances or how much help you got. Only your THINKING changed.

The takeaway? You CAN do this.

"DON'T COMPARE TO THE INCOMPARABLE."

Quoted from the Sunday Times Magazine by Matt Rudd:

"Skimpy, Leggy. Hourglass. Risqué. Enjoying a workout. Hits the beach just two months after giving birth ... Arrrgggghhhh. This week, I have been surfing many celebrity websites. And for the good of humanity/sanity, I would like all of the above word/phrases expunged from the Internet forthwith. Along with 'spills into'. And 'steamy'. And 'how does she do it?' Because she doesn't. Someone else does it for her."

Yes indeed. PTs and chefs, yoga retreats in Ibiza, a full time nanny, and that's before they airbrush the picture.

Real women aren't Barbies, and who on earth would want to be one in reality? These women aren't even necessarily happy with their lot anyway.

Healthy is great. Perfect is ... well, non-existent actually.

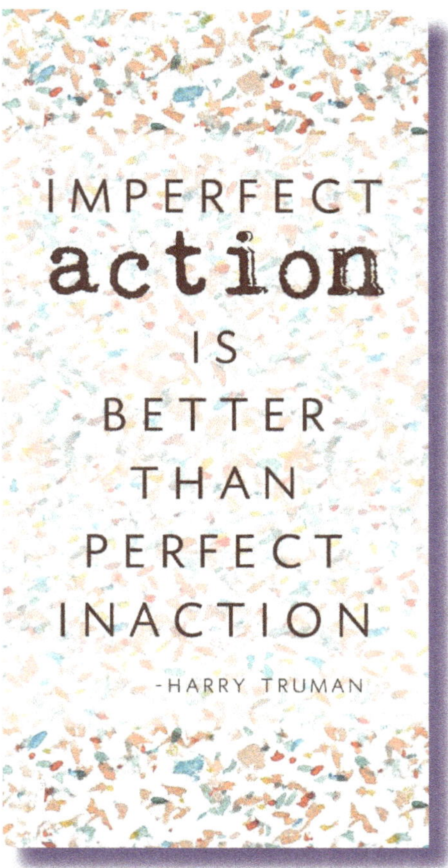

Available to you is all the information and resources you will ever need to reach your goal weight, tone up, have more energy and repair your relationship with food. But none of it means anything if you're spending all your time reading and learning, leaving no time for doing.

Of course I want all of you to be educated and empowered so you know exactly what you need to do to stay healthy and feel your best forever. But you've got to ACT on it too!

Are you eating Fit Mum style today?

Have you got a workout planned today or this week?

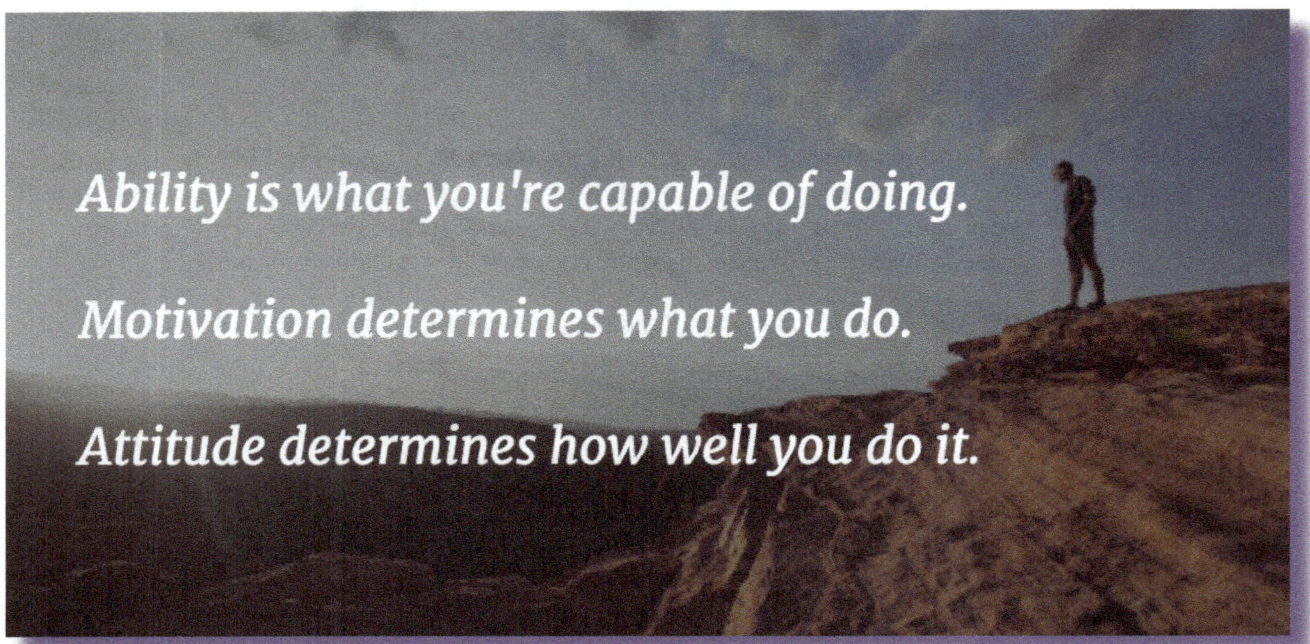

The first is my responsibility, the second is both ours, and the third is yours.

Ability. I need to provide you with the correct and relevant information for you to be able to take action on it and make changes.

Motivation. I will try and motivate and encourage you in every way I know how, but I'm not with you 24/7 and there will certainly be times when your motivation is low, and when you need to try and get yourself motivated. If in doubt, ask: "What would Polly do?"

Attitude. I can't force you to do a workout, I can't make your meals for you, I can't dictate your every minute. You have all the tools and resources you need at your disposal, but ultimately you have to be the one who does it. What results do you want? How much do you want them? Are you prepared to do what needs to be done to get them?

I'm here to help and guide you every step of the way, but it's a team effort. Teamwork will always be better than attempting things on your/my own!

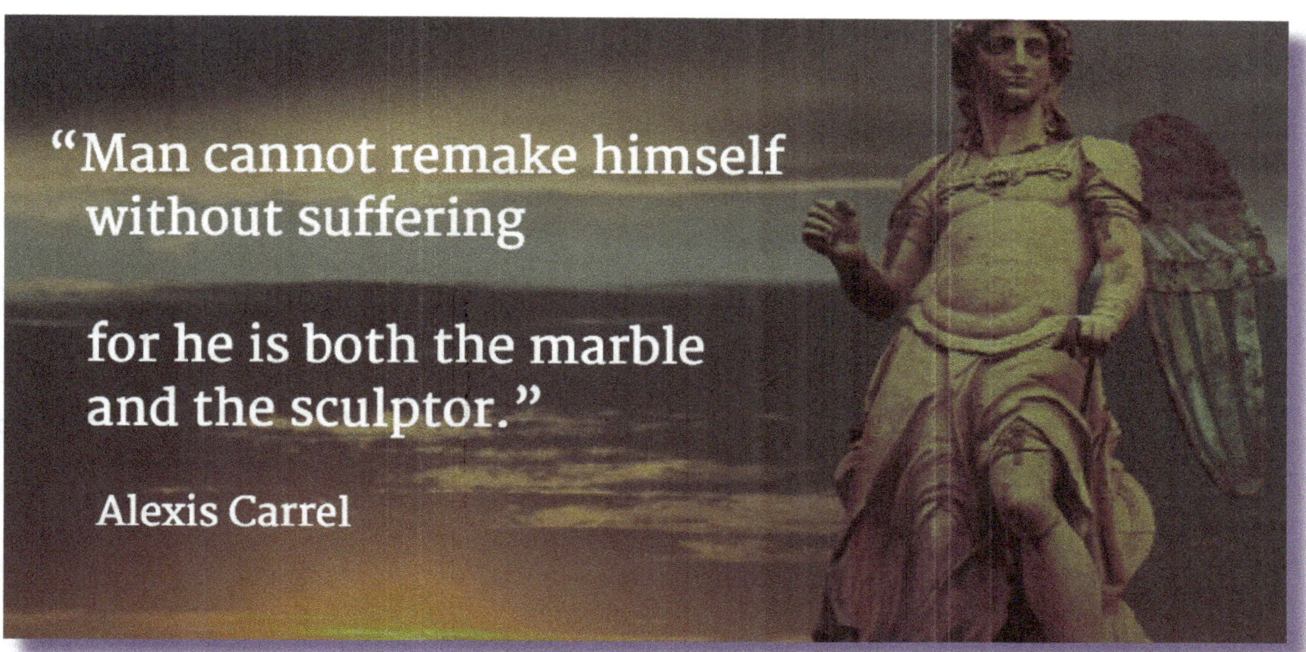

A mistake that drives people to 'quick fixes', 'fads' and, of course, giving up, is the idea that everything will always be easy.

The first time you got behind the wheel of a car was not easy. In fact it was scary, confusing, took a lot of time and energy. Now? You do it without thinking.

When learning any new skill – and yes, making exercise and healthy eating a natural and easy part of your life is a skill – will not come overnight. It will be a challenge at first. But the more you do it, the easier it gets, and at some point (which is different for everyone) it will become natural, just 'the way you do things'.

Yes, you still have to pay attention to the road, always; and watch the traffic lights, always; and be mindful of the speed limit, always. And you will 'always' need to think a little bit to avoid a food-crash. But for the most part, after a while, things will feel a lot more on autopilot!

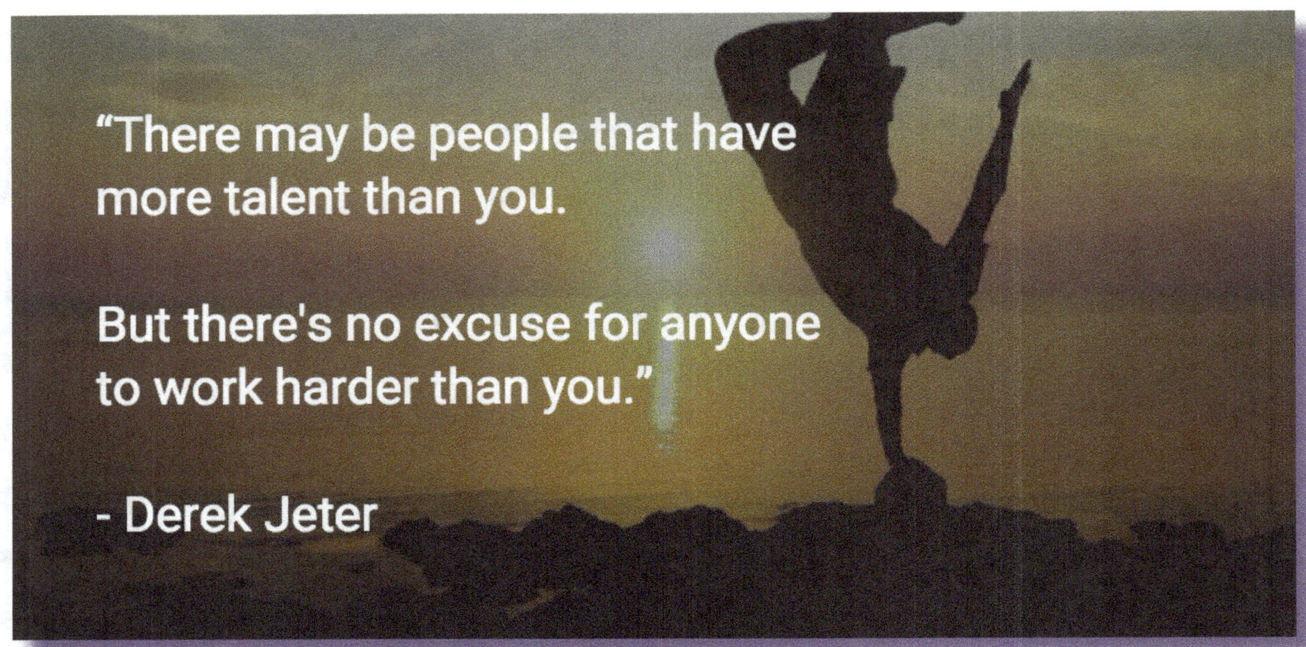

Turn on the telly, there's the Olympic medallists.

Flick through Instagram, there's those skinny Insta-'models' with their perfect bodies and perfect (supposedly anyway) lives.

At the school gates, there's 'that' Mum who always looks so polished and in control.

Look, we don't all have 24/7 home help/chefs/trainers/etc./etc. and yes, sometimes talent and genetics do play a part. But nobody was 'successful' without working damn hard at their 'skill', whether that be winning races or looking hot on the beach.

In fact actions and choices are massive in comparison to genetics. I've worked with a sports genetics company who know that to win an Olympic medal you need to work hard for years, training. To win a GOLD medal you need the right genes; no Gold sprinter doesn't have the right genes, as far as has been tested. But you can still get to the Olympics (metaphorically, obviously!). You can absolutely reach your goals if you're prepared to go for them.

Have you ever stopped 'trying' because you thought a goal was out of your reach?

Is that thought still holding you back now?

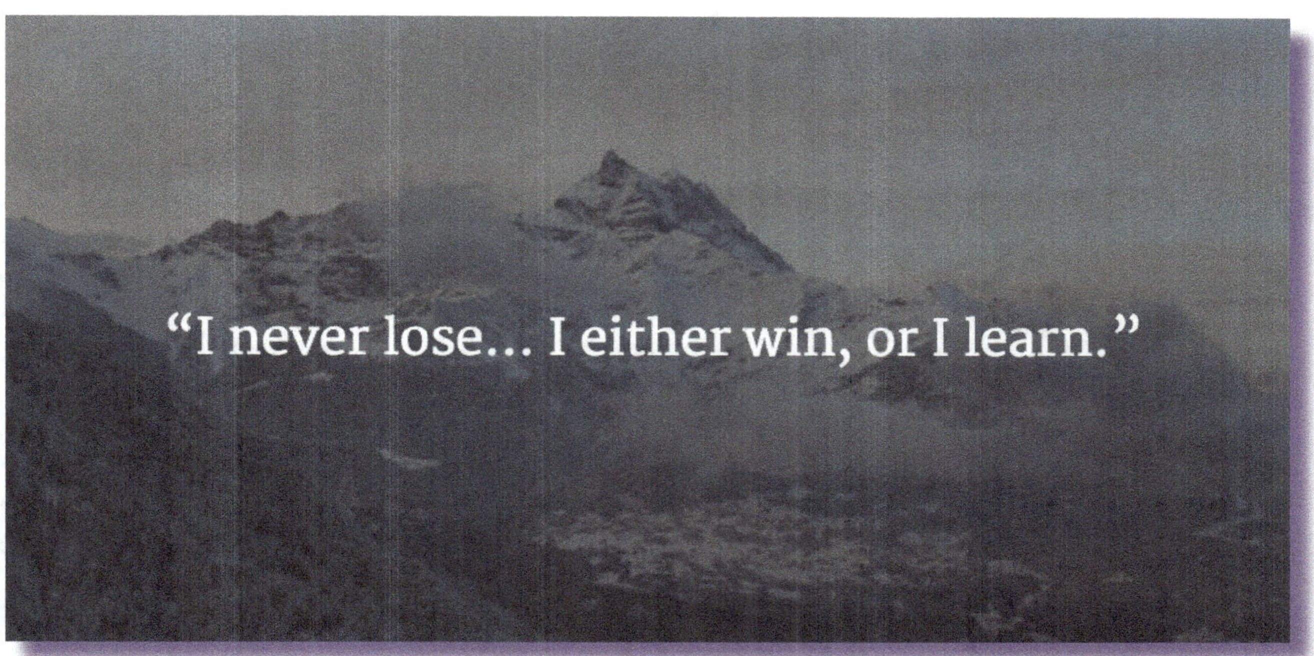

This is what your weight loss journey with The Fit Mum Formula is about, learning what works for YOU.

Had serious cravings that led to eating half a cake? What caused those cravings?

So hungry you ate all hubby's chips too? Why did your own food intake not satisfy you?

So tired by Friday evening you ordered takeaway, all six dishes of it. What was going on in the lead up to the evening?

AND MORE IMPORTANTLY ....

What can you learn from each of these events and can change in future to prevent them happening again?

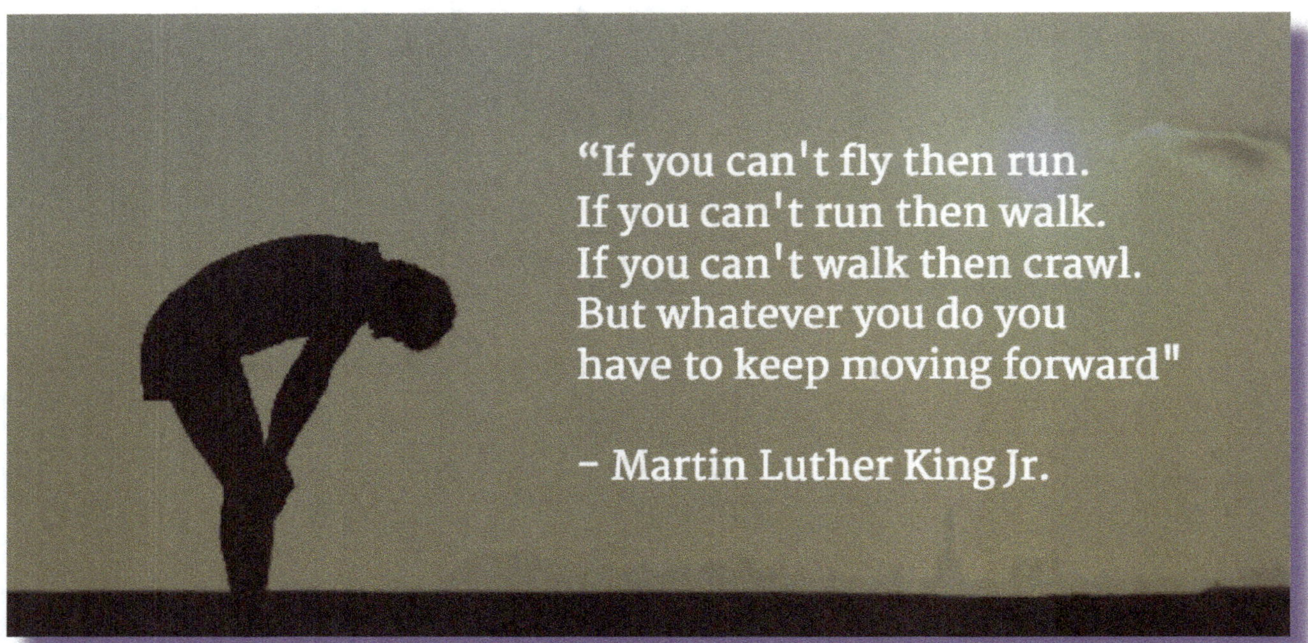

Ever have a bad day when you just want to give up?

We all do right? Not just with diet and exercise but in life in general. But giving up is the worst thing you can do as all momentum comes to a halt.

Sometimes you have to slow down, scale back, simplify things with smaller goals, but don't stop moving forward.

How do you keep going when you want to give up?

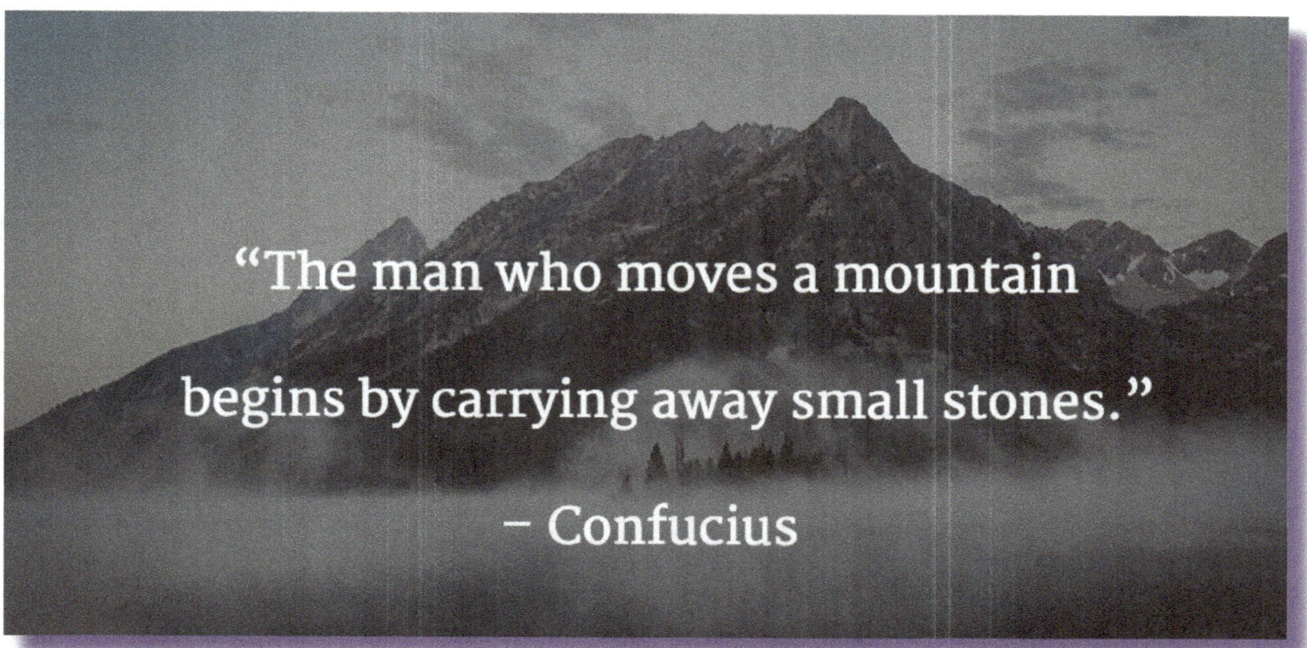

It's only overwhelming if you let it.

The other quote I love is, "How do you eat an elephant? One bite at a time".

Don't think about overhauling everything you know at once. That's far too much to take in. It can work (so by all means give it a go), but usually leads to getting confused, overburdened and disheartened when you 'fail' to get everything perfect.

A much more likely strategy for most people is to work on improving one thing at a time, a thing small enough that you are unlikely to fail. Maybe it's just getting breakfast right and doing one workout on a weekend. Then from there you can add in a second workout during the week, and perhaps a healthy evening meal.

Suddenly it all feels a lot more do-able, and a lot less give-up-able!

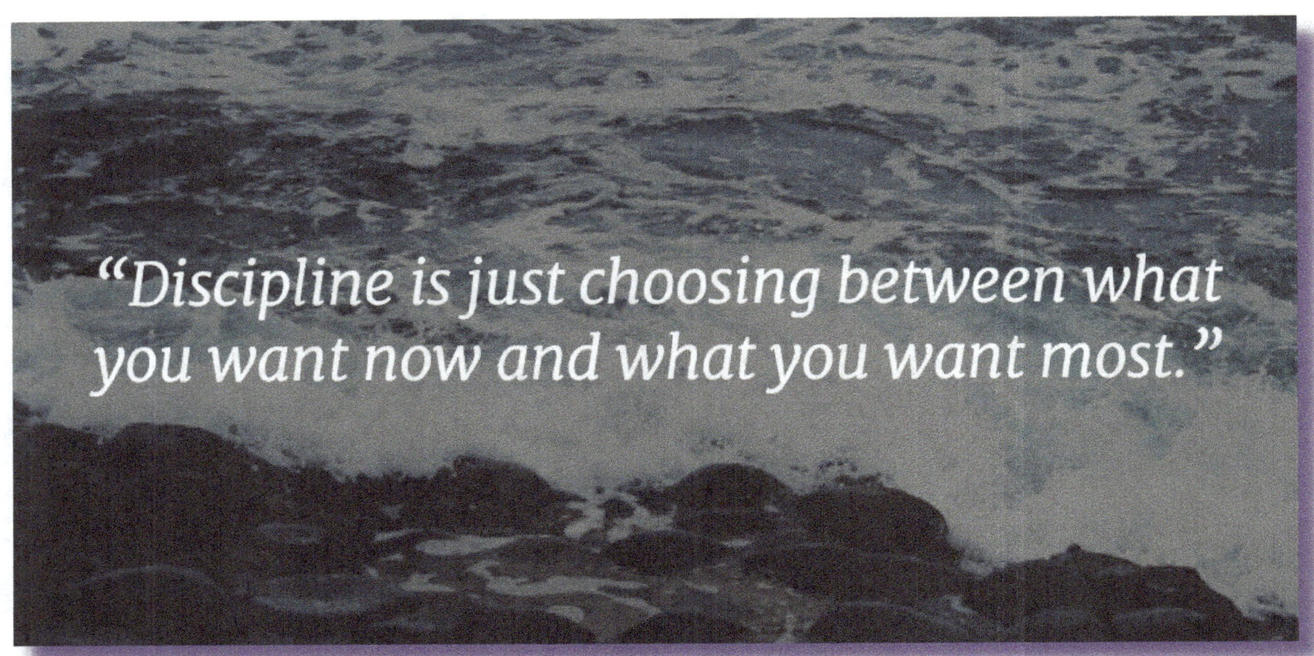

It's a simple thing you can do every time you are tempted to do something unhelpful, like have a double Mr Whippy with flake, sauce and marshmallows, instead of a small tub then grab an apple when you get home (or whatever).

Ask yourself, "What do I want more? This ice cream? Or to feel happy with my body, confident in skimpier clothes this summer, and pride in myself for having the strength to carry out good intentions?" The last one is incredibly motivating; it gives you the self-belief that you CAN do this, and so can continue to do so.

What do YOU want most? I LOVE ice cream, but not so much that I'm prepared to sacrifice feeling awesome by eating half a tub in one go. I'll stick to the occasional small treat (or healthy Greek yoghurt alternative – win, win)!

"IS WHO YOU WANT TO BE, WHO YOU REALLY WANT TO BE?"

Who are you trying to beat?

Who are you comparing yourself to?

Who do you want to look like?

There's a race, called the Self-Transcendence Race, and it is 3,100 miles long. It's the longest foot race on earth. For comparison's sake, a marathon (which most people will never do) is 26 miles.

Lesson?

There will ALWAYS be someone better, faster, fitter, slimmer, prettier, more toned than you. If someone being 'better' than you makes you feel bad, 'less than', or like you'll never be 'good enough', you're in for a life of misery.

There is nobody quite like you. You are special and unique in your own ways and while someone else might be 'better' in some areas, I guarantee they fall short elsewhere. Your best qualities are just different to their best ones.

I would rather my 'best' qualities weren't as superficial as winning something like 'rear of the year' anyway, quite frankly!

As an old woman, will you be sad you never became an Instagram model? Or will you look at the legacy you left behind – a growing family, friends you made smile, experiences you created.

Health and your body is important, but it's not the only thing that's important.

"INACTION IS EASY. ACTION IS HARD."

That's why you stay stuck, it's easy!

I've heard that people have to hear something three times before they take action on it.

Maybe in the marketing world where you, say, buy something once, you only have to take action once, so perhaps seeing a pair of shoes three times (magazine, catalogue, shop window) might make you take action. But when it comes to things we need to do every day, several times a day (like eat, for example), it's going to take more than three times thinking about or seeing healthy food for it to become a daily habit.

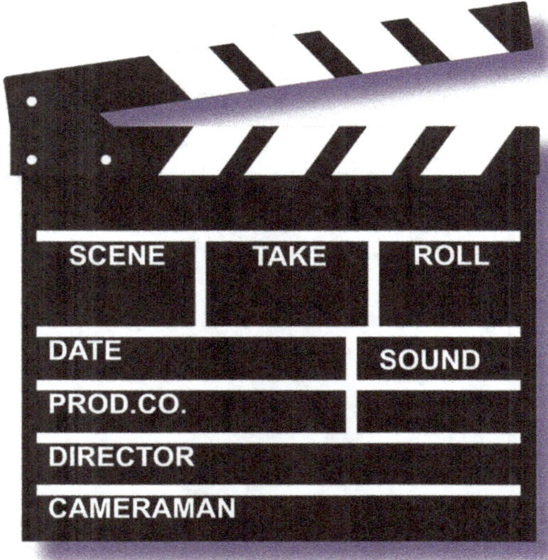

It has to be done day in, day out, with effort, until one day it starts happening naturally. But it starts with moving on from thinking about it to doing it. Action.

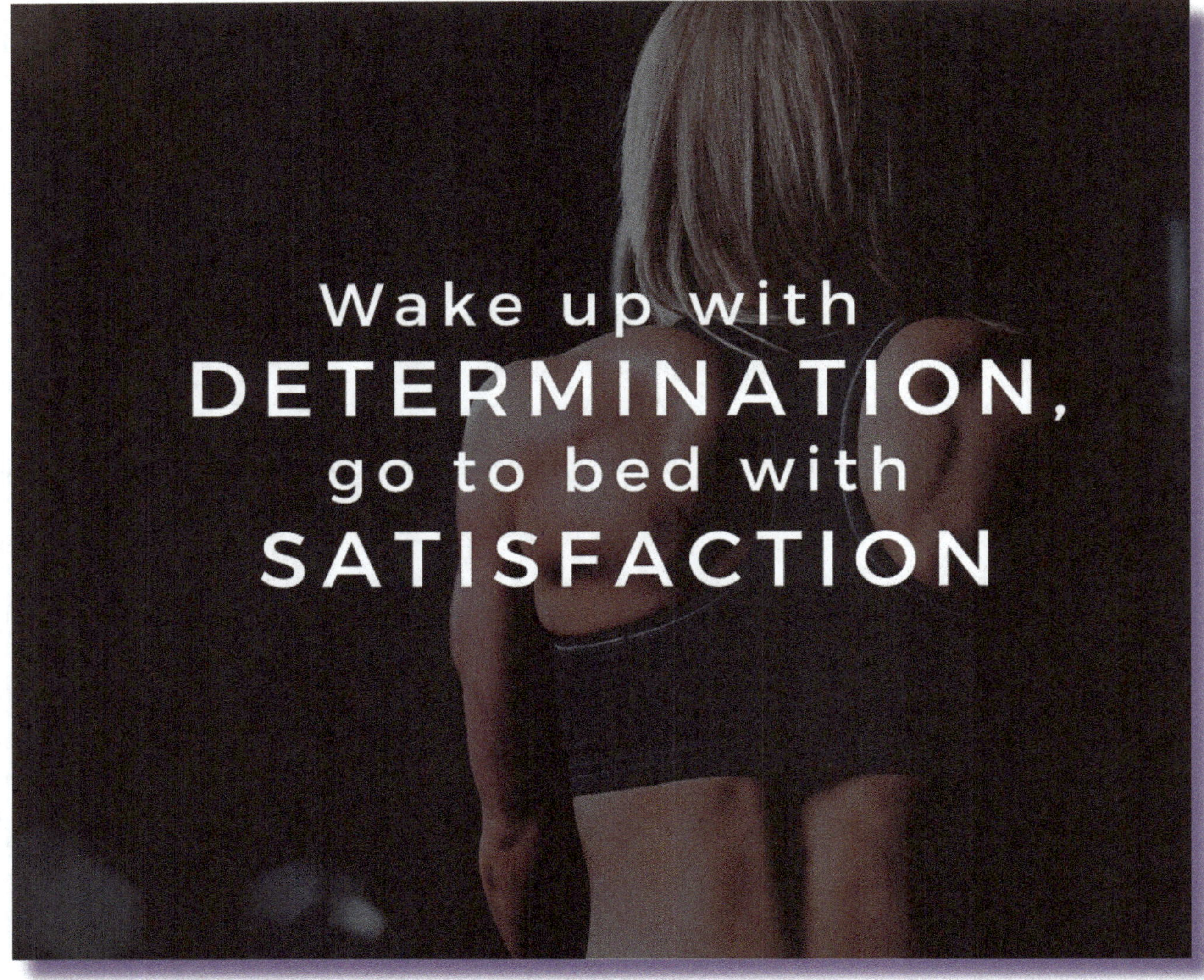

Have you ever felt REALLY determined to succeed at something?

Maybe it was an exam you wanted to get a good grade in; a race you wanted to win at school; perhaps it was even giving birth – talking to yourself in a stupor of pain (and/or drugs) – "I CAN DO THIS!"

Remember how that felt? The adrenaline and passion, the fire in your belly.

Now think of what you want to achieve in terms of having a body you are proud of, having boundless energy and a love for life, with you feeling confident at the centre of it.

Now put the two together. Feel that determination and passion and do what it takes to get that body confidence back!

What will you do this week to get closer to your goals?

DO IT NOW, SOMETIMES 'LATER' BECOMES 'NEVER'

Who here suffers from procrastination?

I'm normally pretty focused, but if I'm tired or have brain fog (too much gluten and dairy, or not enough sleep does this to me) or have been in front of the computer too long, that's when I start faffing and putting things off.

I find staying one step ahead of these 'moods' stops them from getting the better of me. I've already got my workout things out and ready for tomorrow morning, I'm not going to let 'might be late for school' be an excuse, just because I've not got myself organised.

How do you motivate yourself into doing things you 'should' be doing?

"IT'S ALL IN YOUR ... TUMMY."

The mind–belly connection.

How often do you feel stressed, annoyed, under pressure, upset or lonely? I'm sure you feel at least one at some point every day. And that's fine, these are NORMAL feelings and part of life. It's how we react to these which matters.

Next time you feel one of the above (or similar), tune into your body and notice what happens.

Does your heart rate increase?

Do you get knots in your stomach?

Do you feel hungry or feel like you can't eat?

Do you have an urge for chocolate or another food, or perhaps it's wine?

Being aware of this may give you insight into why you eat certain things at certain times, even when you don't 'need' them. Or alternatively, not eat only to eat too much later instead.

Try it and take note of what you notice.

"ARE YOUR GOALS SMART?
ARE YOU EVEN SETTING GOALS?"

Not everyone needs to (if you're good at staying consistent and on track, and are making progress, then you're probably OK).

If, however, you need a more concrete plan, try creating your own SMART goals:

S: Specific, e.g., I want to be size X by my summer holiday.

M: Measurable, e.g. I will know I'm making progress by measuring myself and charting it on my TFMF progress charts (provided in the next chapter).

A: Achievable. If you're 6 ft. tall you're never going to be a size 8 (or you shouldn't be).

R: Realistic. The goal you have set is realistic for the time allowed (no 'lose 2 stone in a week' goals please!)

T: Timely. Work out how much you need to lose week by week, depending on how long you're giving yourself and what your goal is (check R again), and measure along the way to make sure you're on track.

Try writing your own SMART goals and post them on social media or tell your friends. Because telling people about your goals is another effective trick – it keeps you accountable!

"WHAT'S REALLY STOPPING YOU LOSING WEIGHT?"

Let's face it, all the information you'll ever need is available on the Internet.

It's not a lack of knowledge problem.

What makes having a coach different? Is it accountability?

Someone to turn to for advice and support?

Someone to reassure you and lift you up when you're having a bad day?

It's never just about the food. If it was then any cut out magazine meal plan would work.

What is YOUR 'not about the food' barrier?

"WHEN THE PAIN OF WHERE YOU ARE BECOMES GREATER THAN THE PAIN OF WHERE YOU WANT TO BE."

They say you will change when the pain of where you are becomes greater than the pain of where you want to be, or the process of getting there.

Change is hard. Change can be painful.

Staying the same, no change, is easy, and not so painful.

And this is why people get stuck. Even if it's in a situation they're not entirely happy with.

Change is scary. But it's always worth it in the end.

Have you gone through a painful, difficult or scary process to reach a goal?

Overcoming an eating disorder was the scariest, most difficult thing I have ever done, and I would not have done it without seeking professional support. But it was worth every scary difficult painful moment.

I am stronger because I had to be.
I'm smarter because of my mistakes,
happier because I've known sadness
and wiser from all of my lessons.

This sums up the way I help you get your health, food and body back in your control.

There is no such thing as getting it wrong, failing or doing things badly.

There are only lessons, which means you can learn from them.

Tomorrow you are a wiser, smarter, more experienced person than you were yesterday.

Sometimes those lessons have to be learnt the hard way!

Can't stop at one chocolate from a sharing pack? Maybe individually wrapped ones are better for now.

Skipped lunch but picked at junk all afternoon? You've learnt skipping meals doesn't work.

What have you learnt this week? I still learn every day. It's a never-ending process.

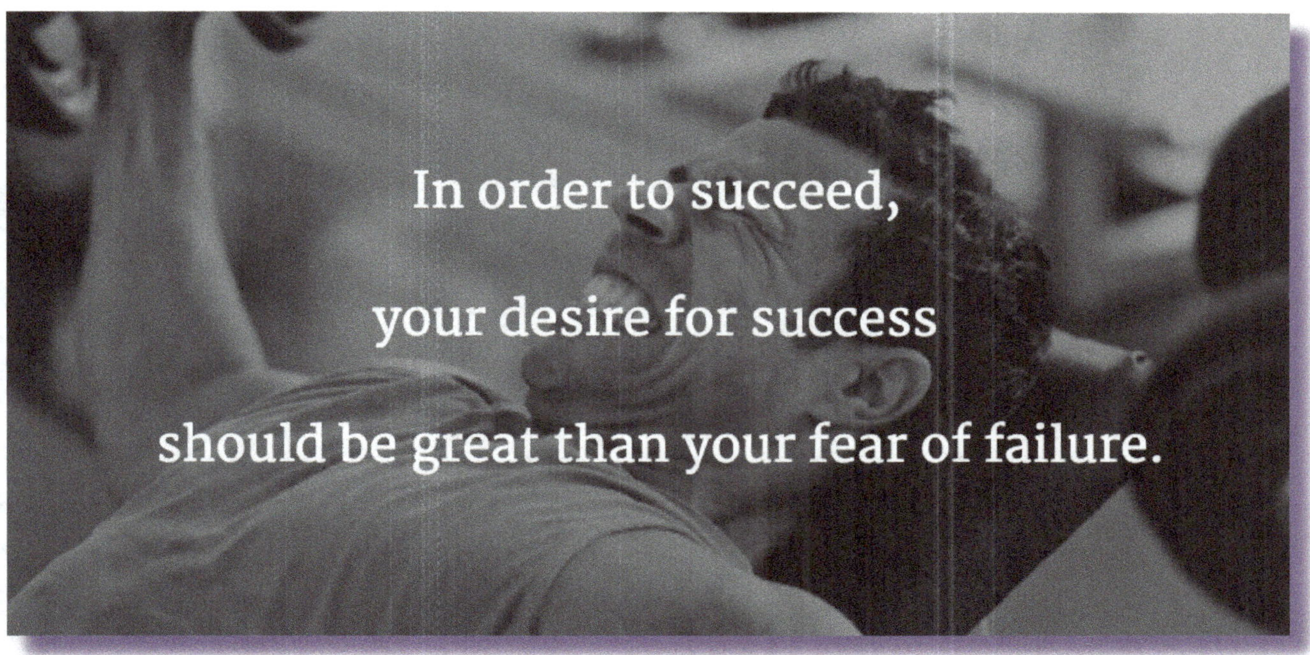

You will do what you need to do when the pain of where you're at becomes greater than the pain of change. Change is painful and scary. Staying put is easy. But it's also holding you back from a world of opportunity and happiness.

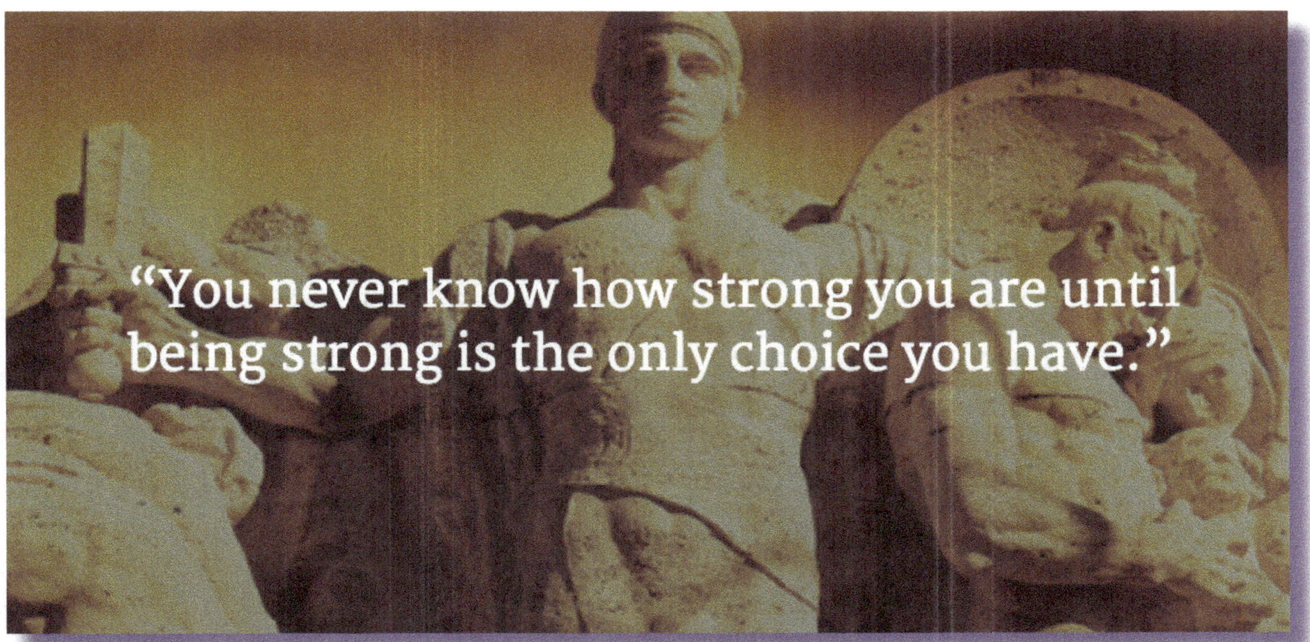

Whatever it is, you CAN do it. That strength is in there somewhere.

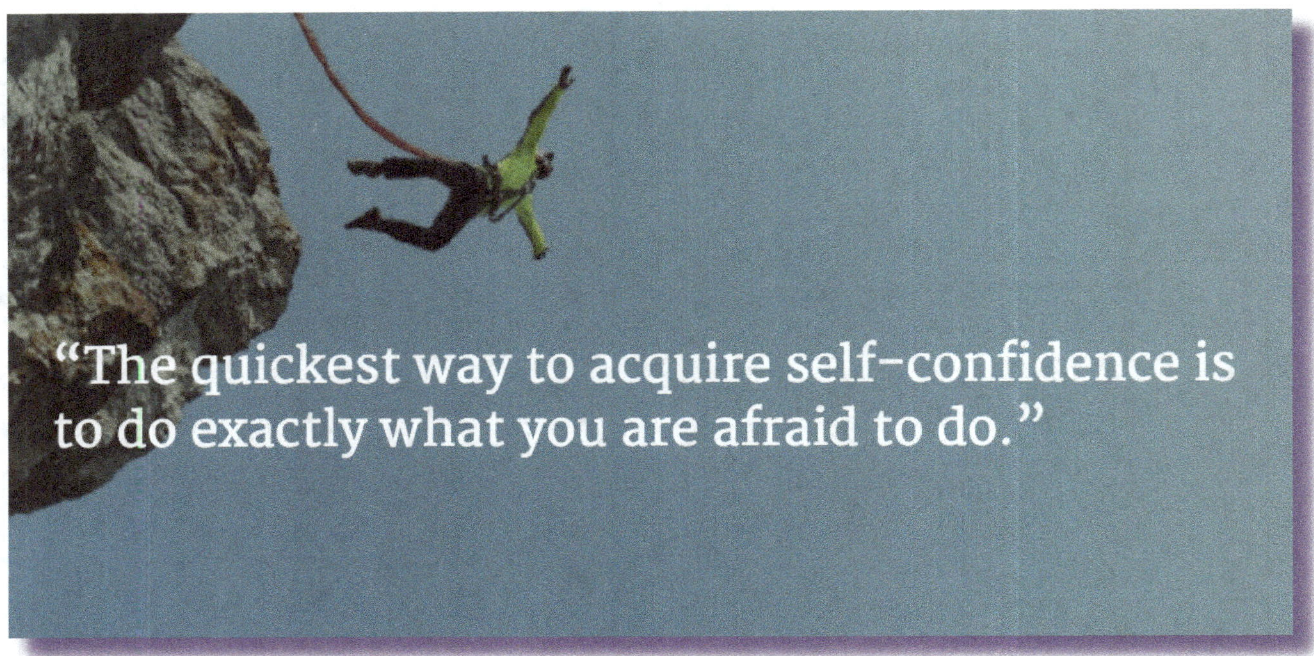

What will you do today that's scary?

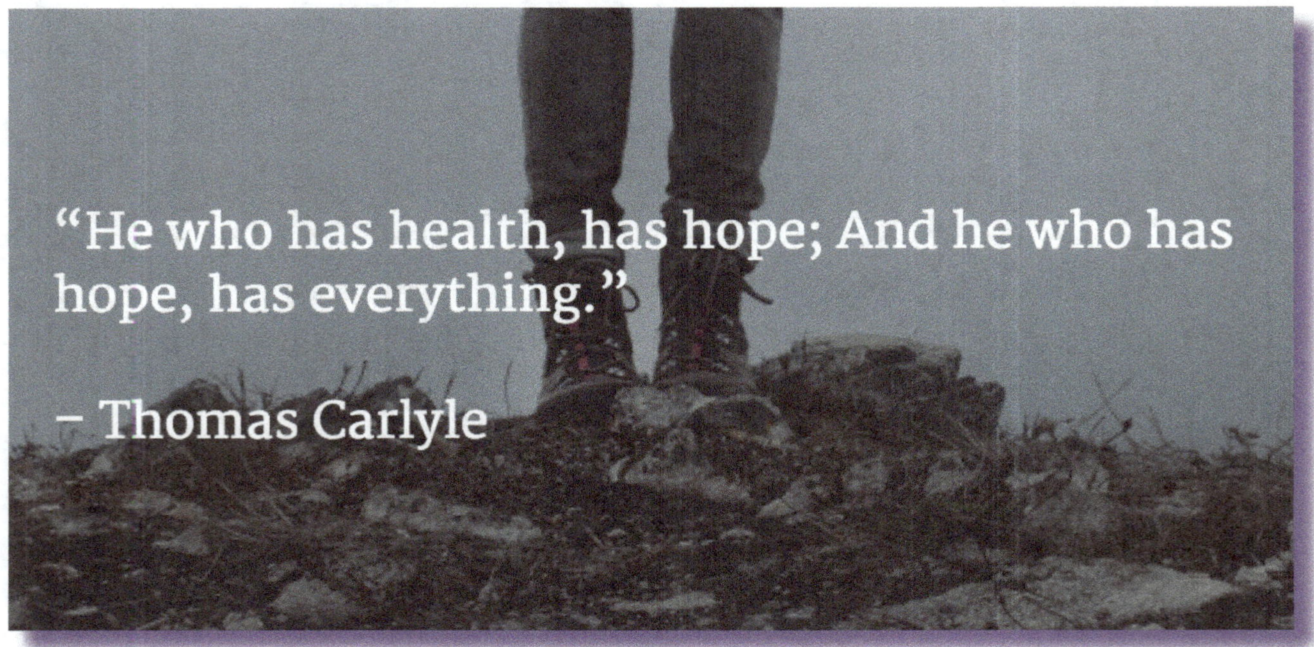

Want more happiness? Improving your physical health is a good place to start.

And I don't mean just to look good.

A healthy body is a healthy mind.

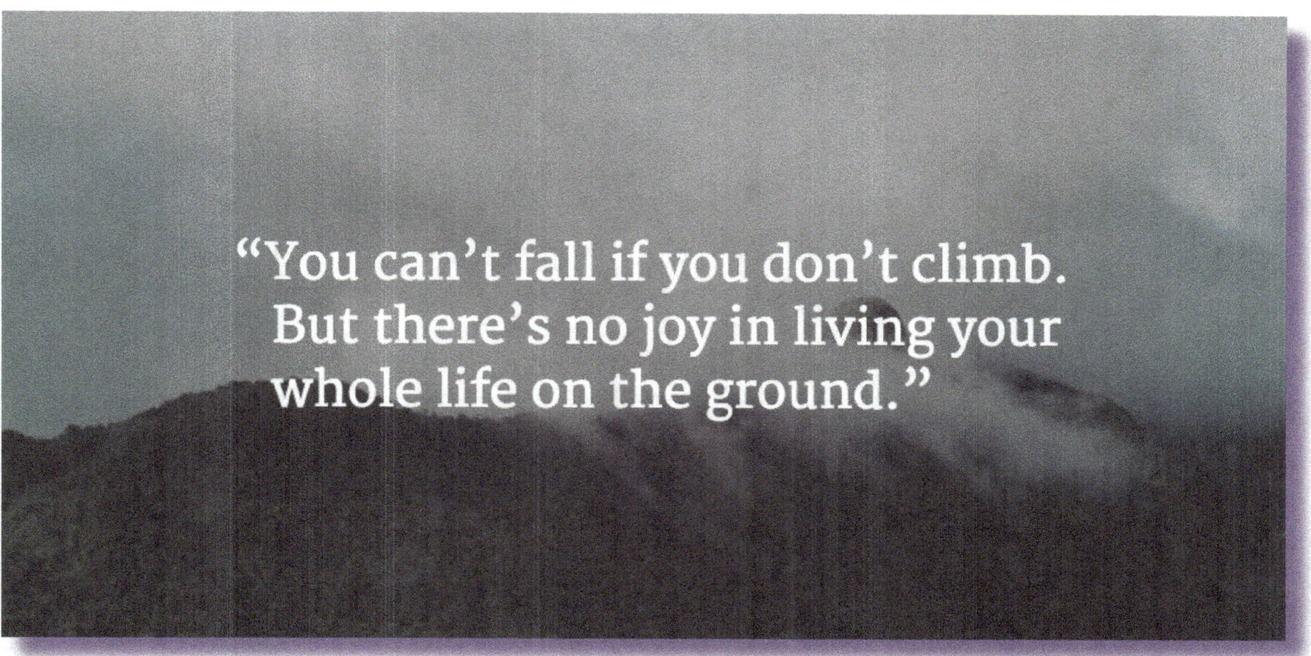

Live each day for the moment. Take a risk. The worst that could happen won't be nearly as bad as you think.

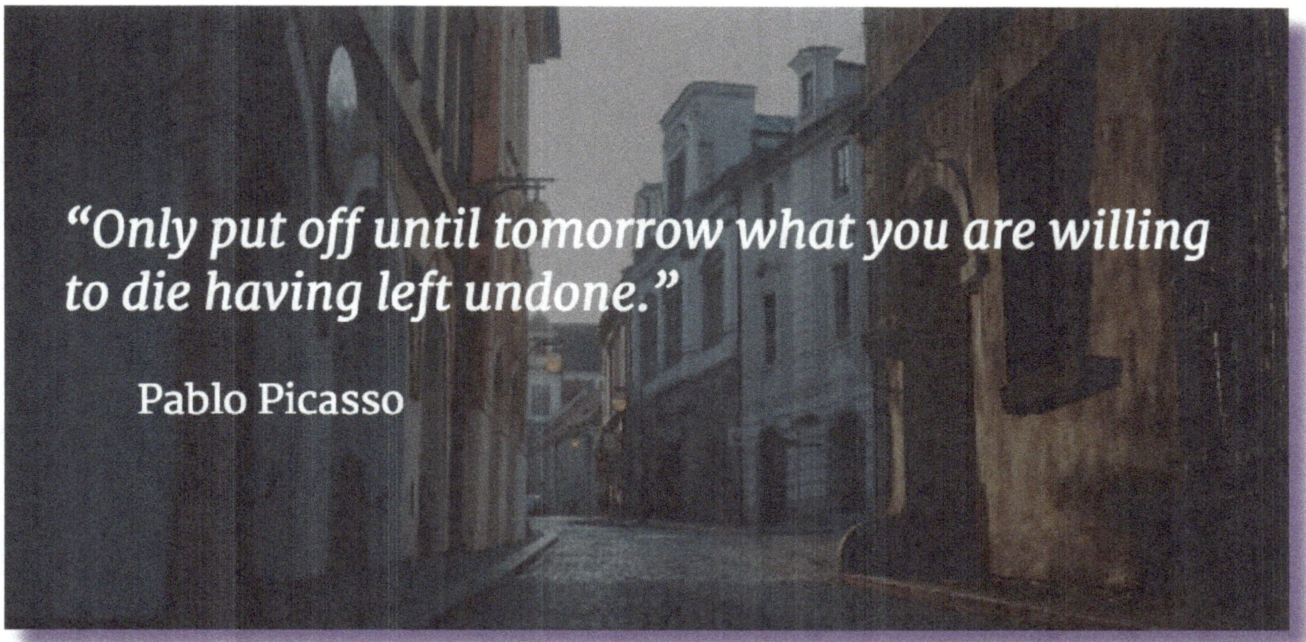

Live for today, it won't be repeated.

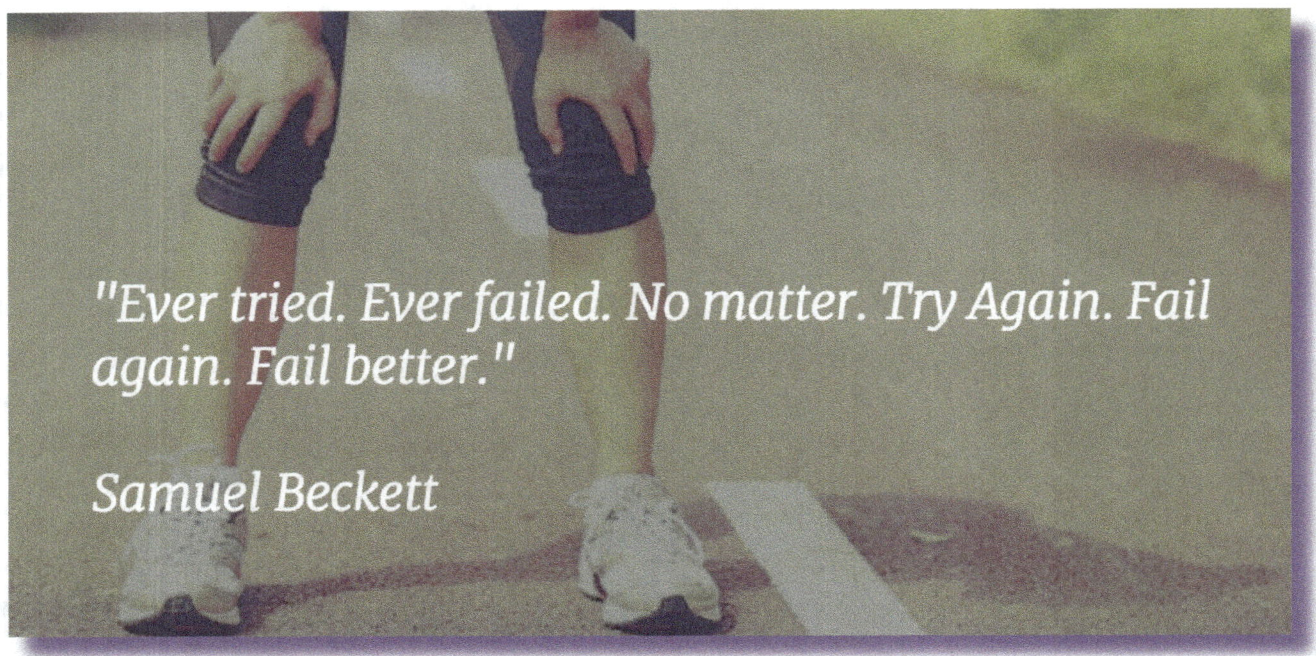

Everything in life is a lesson. There are no failures in life, only lessons.

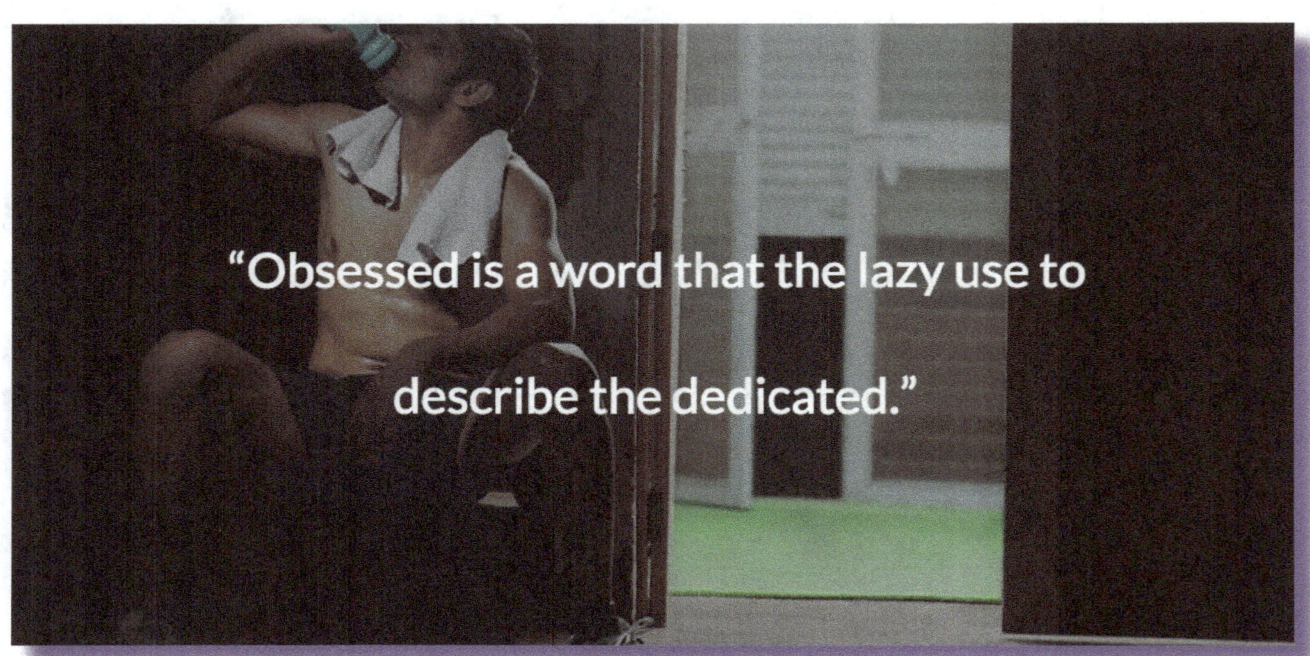

I am officially obsessed and dedicated to chocolate. Just kidding (sort of). But high quality cocoa and dark chocolate makes my body feel food and perform well, and that is something I am dedicated to.

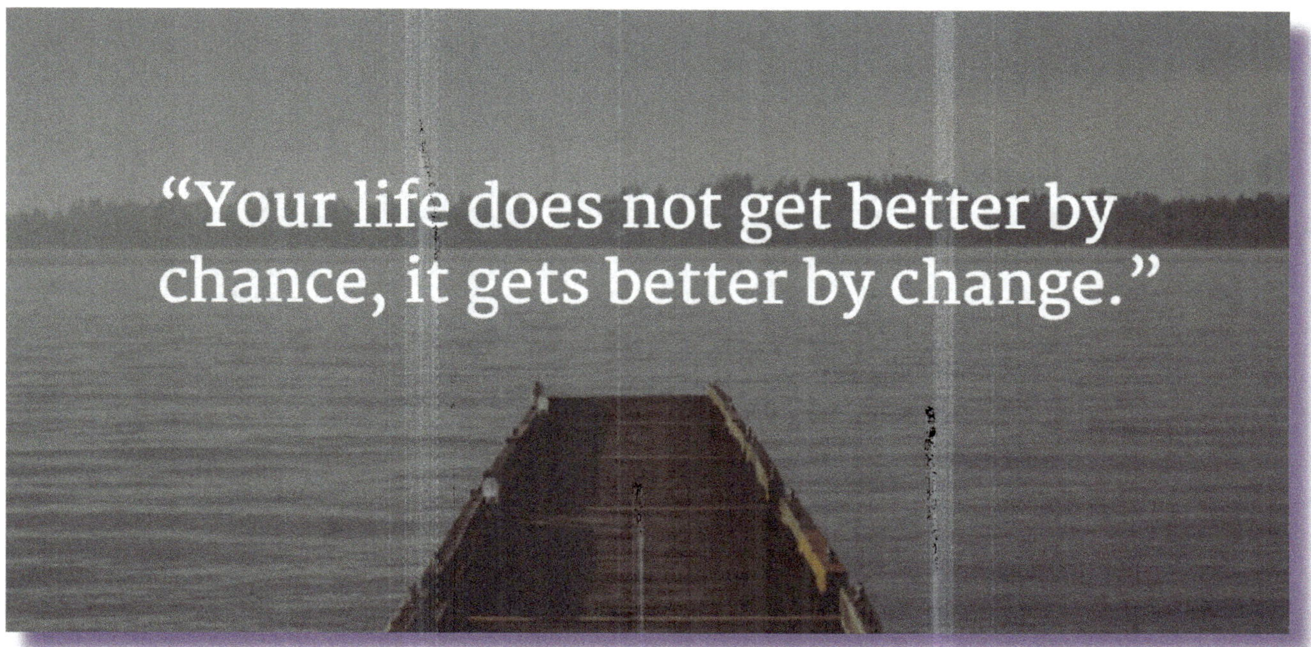

Action beats perfection every time.

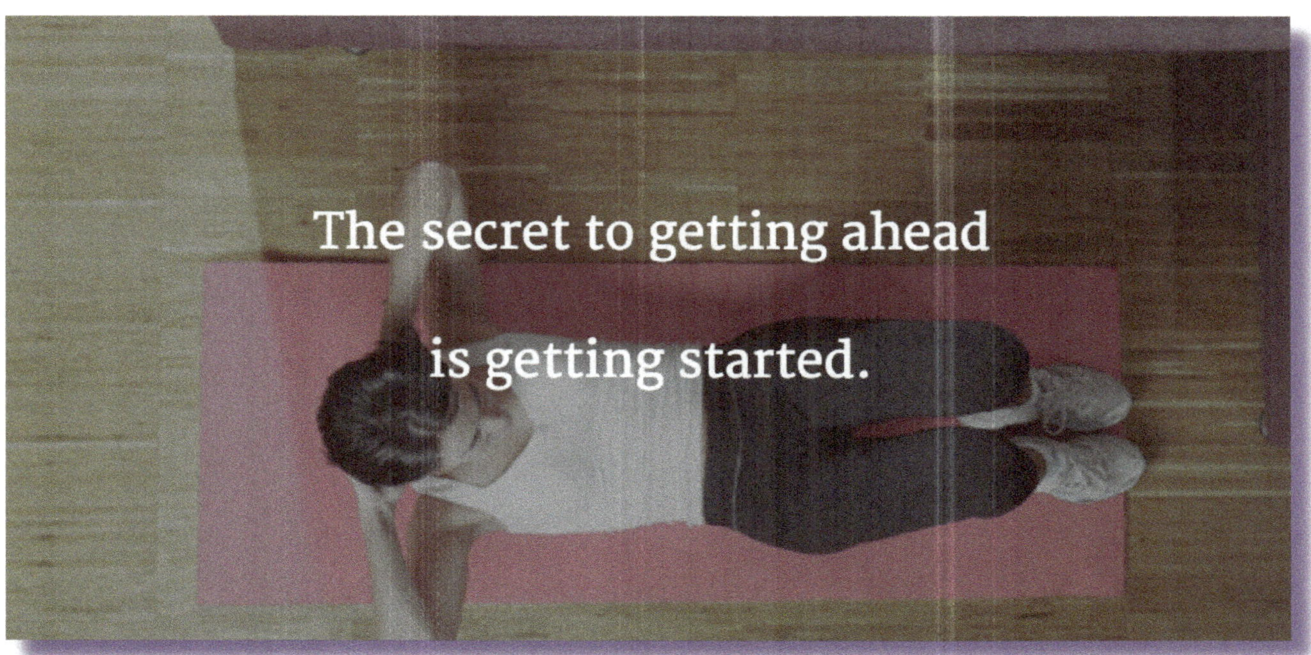

I wrote this on a Monday. But you don't have to wait until Monday to 'start'.

Start now, and this time don't quit.

> Your future self is watching you right now through memories.
>
> Do yourself a favour and make it something worth watching.

What would the movie of your life look like?

"THE BEST WAY TO GET STARTED IS TO STOP TALKING AND START DOING."

When you combine Walt Disney with some motivation, that has to be a winner. Don't live your life like it's a cartoon. Live it for real.

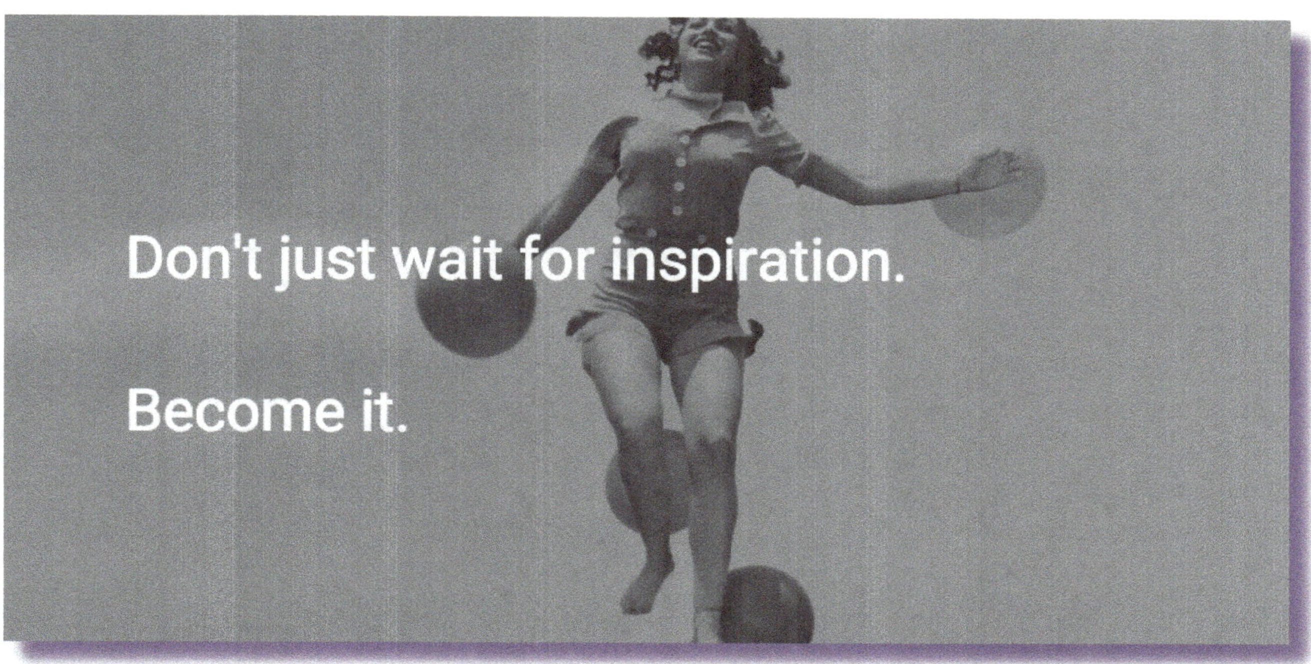

If there's no one to inspire you, create it yourself. Inspire yourself.

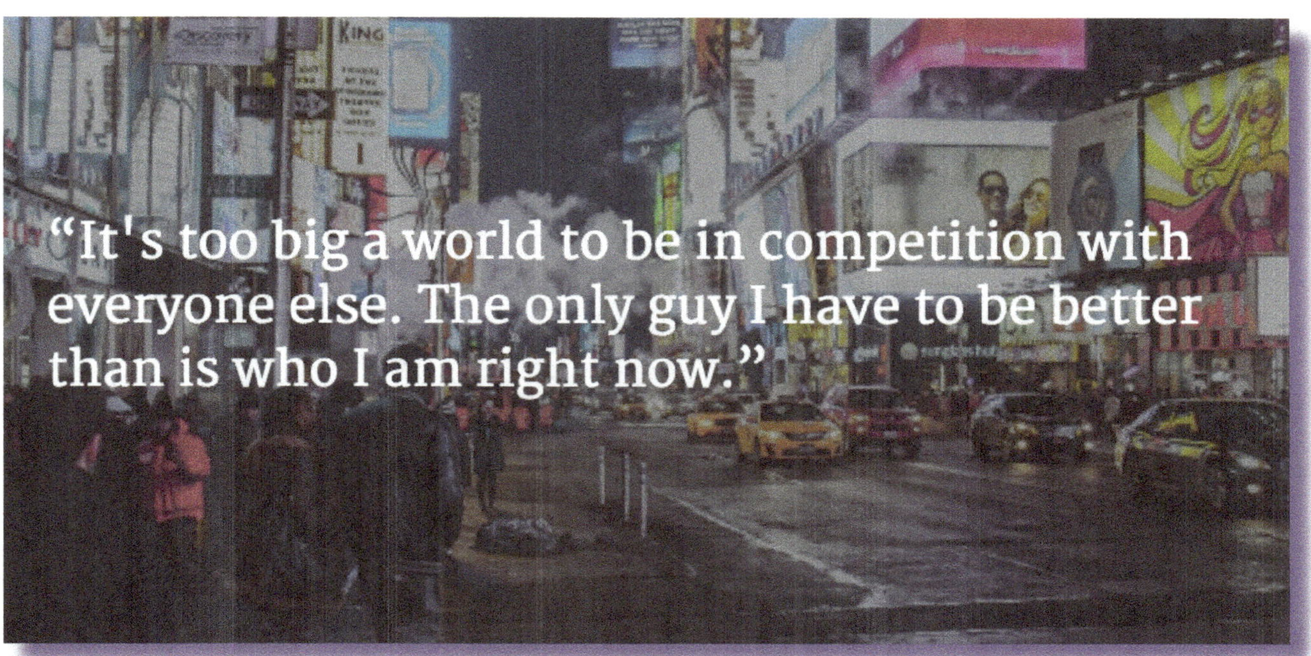

The only person you need to beat is yesterday's you.

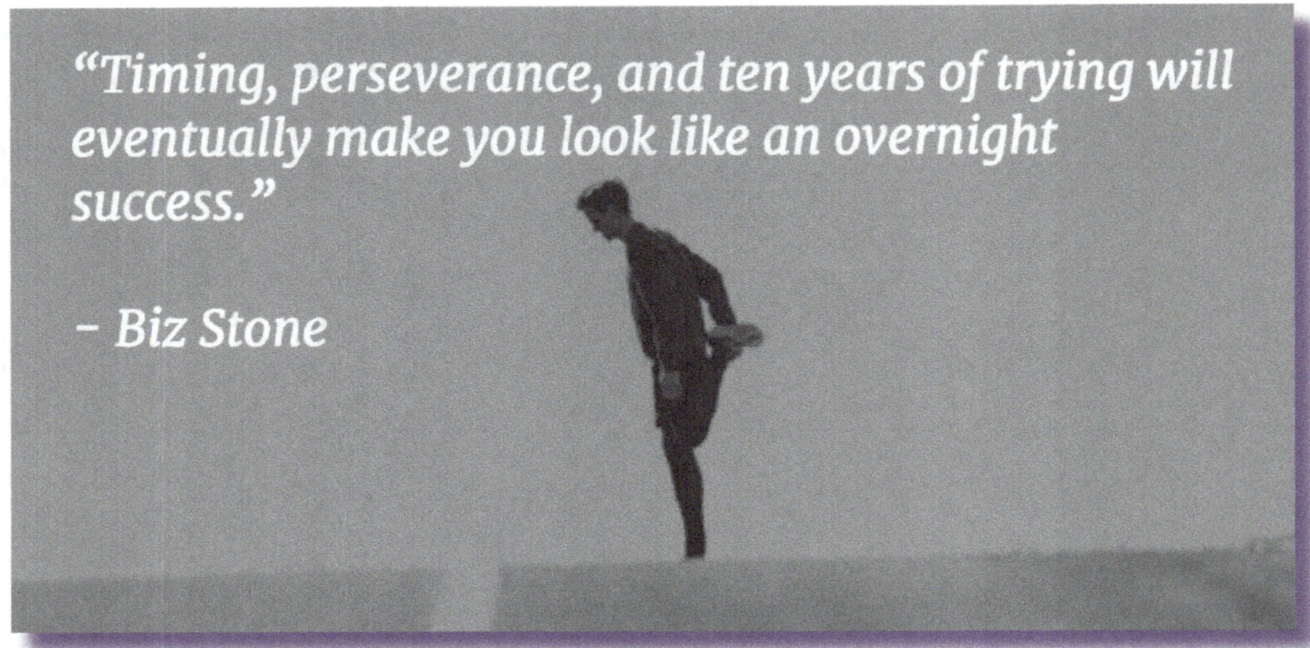

Have you ever tried what you now realise was a 'quick fix' diet in the past?

Probably, if you're like most women.

Did it work? If you regained the weight, in my eyes, it didn't work. Because you didn't learn enough skills to be able to sustain eating well for life.

There is NO quick fix.

There ARE/IS:

- learning to tune into your body and know what it needs

- realising how some choices don't work for you, make life difficult or take you further away from, not closer to, your goals

- killing off old habits that don't help you

- forming new, healthy habits

- learning how to deal with difficult situations rather than using them as an excuse

- being able to bounce back and learn from mistakes, rather than throw in the towel

Rinse and repeat. Rinse and repeat. Rinse and repeat.

This is a journey.

"WHEN YOU'RE 80 YOU'RE GOING TO WISH YOU SPENT MORE TIME LOVING AND APPRECIATING YOUR BODY WHEN YOU WERE 30."

Don't look back in regret, because you spent so much time worrying about your body rather than enjoying it while it's still working.

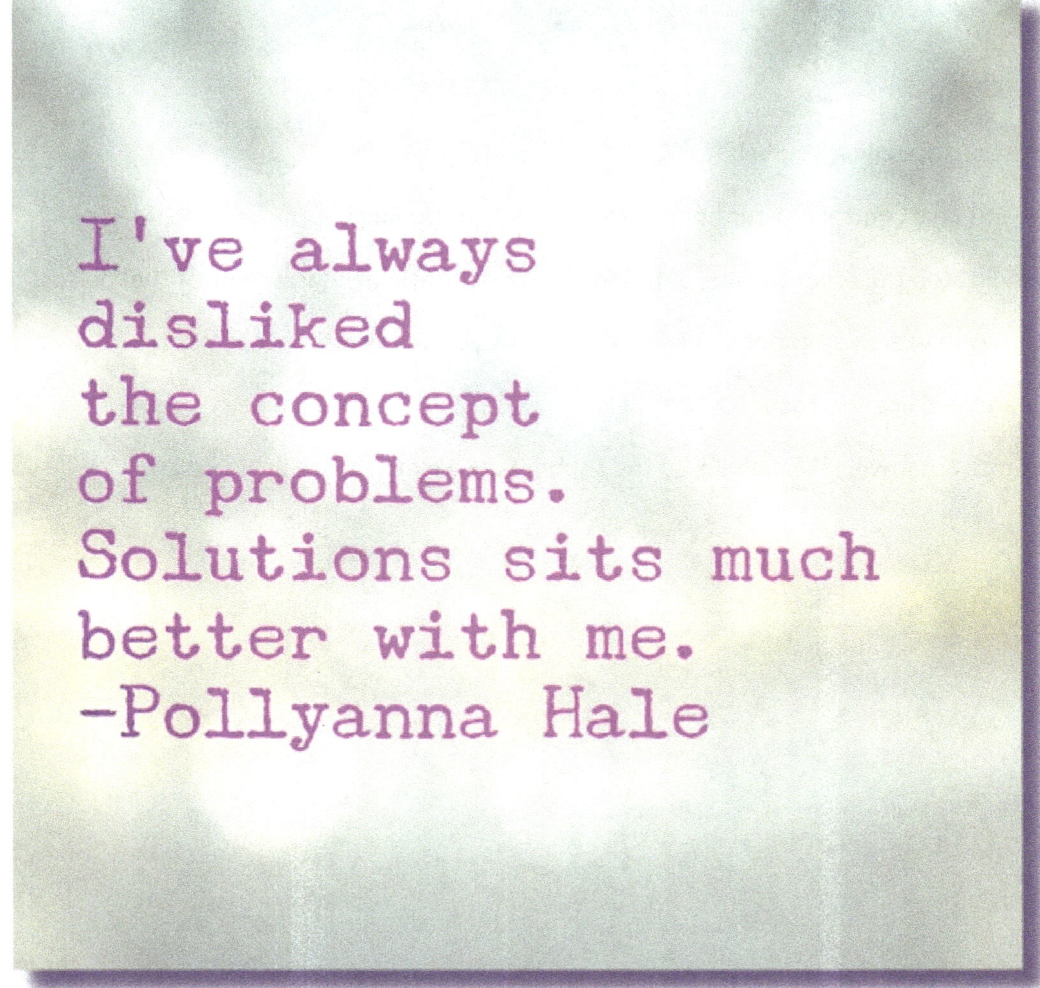

There are very few real problems in life. There are, however, hurdles that need to be overcome. You just need to figure out how.

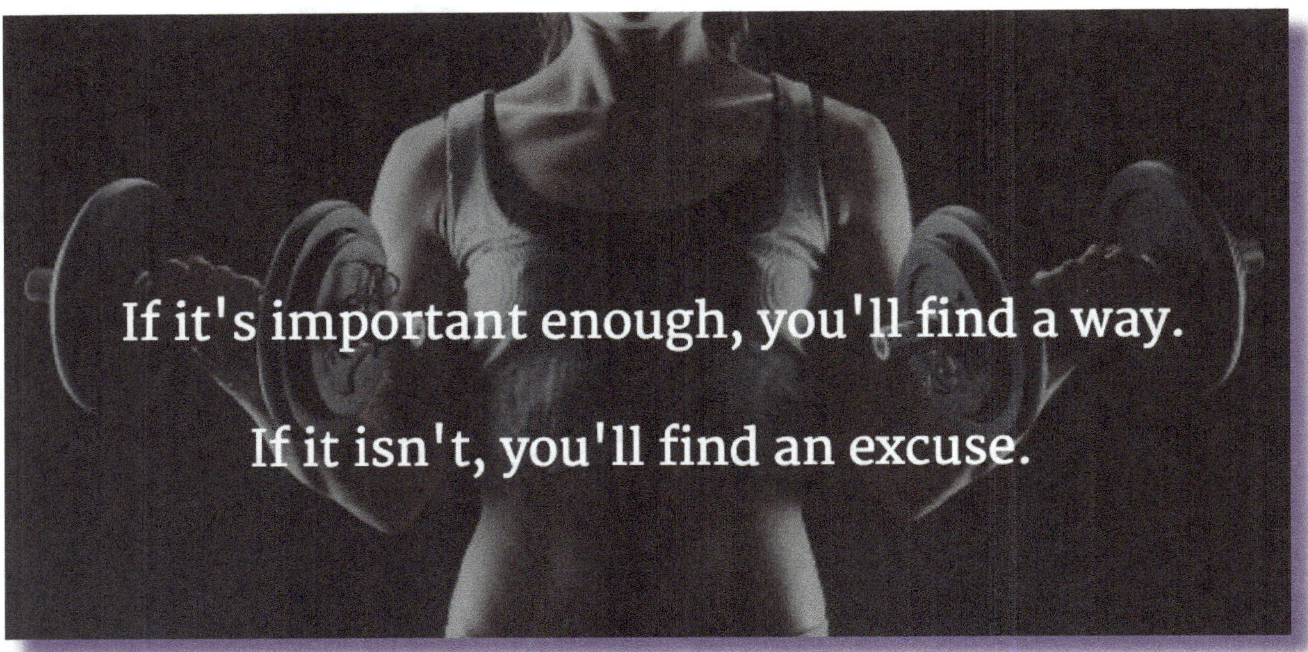

Make today THE day.

- the day you stop telling yourself it's too hard

- the day you take control of your body, rather than it controlling you

- the day you stop the roller coaster of trying one diet after the next in search of the 'perfect' one

- the first day in years you choose to love and care for your body rather than punish it

Want to look and feel like this too?

You can, anytime. But it will take a while, so the sooner you start the better.

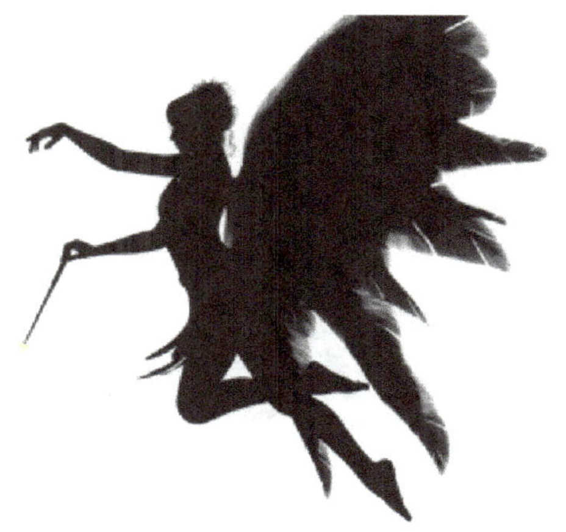

Hello! I'm the fitness fairy. I just sprinkled motivation dust on you. Now go and move your ass. This shit is expensive.

www.thefitmumformula.com

You see, the only thing anyone, including me, can do, is to persuade you to take action on our advice. Don't get me wrong, that's a skill most don't have. But at the end of the day I can't do it for you.

Nobody can, except you.

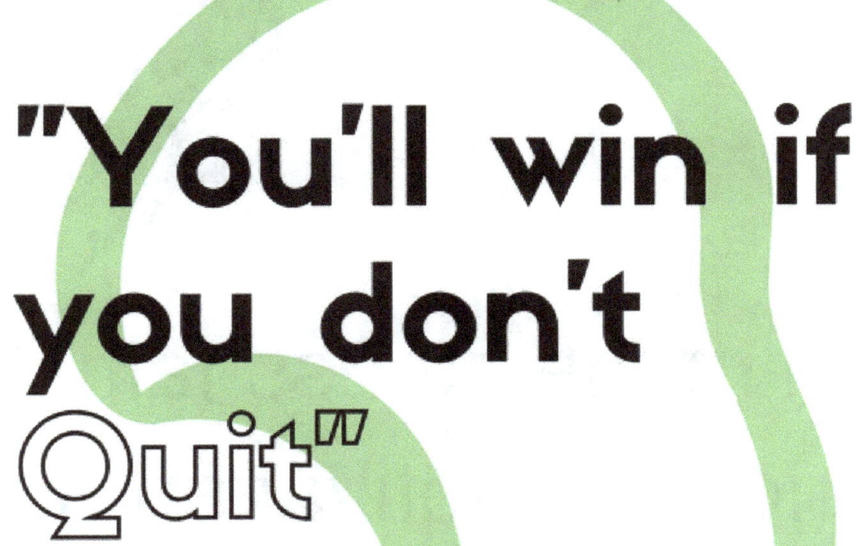

This embodies the BodyBack programme.

You know how it works, no strict meal plans, no 'this and only this works'. You try, you assess, you tweak, assess again. You can't not win!

If something is working for you? Keep doing it.

Not working? Change something, give it enough chance, and then check how/if it's working.

The only way it won't work is if you quit trying to figure out what works.

Of course, I'm always here to help you do that, but the process, nevertheless, is the same. I just help you figure out the answers (and believe me, if there was a one size fits all plan I'd give it to you, there just isn't)!

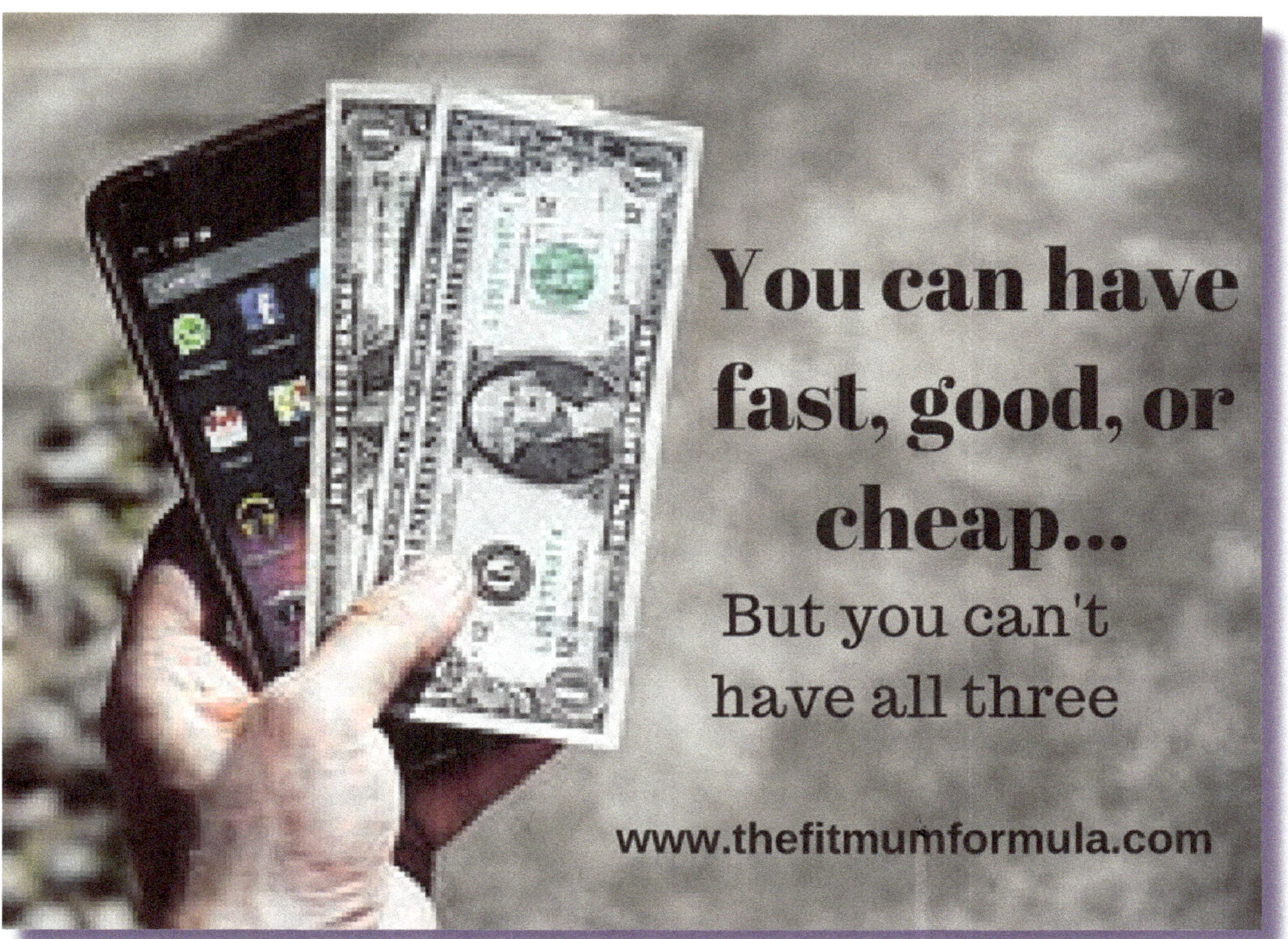

Think about that for a second.

It applies to everything, not just weight loss programmes.

Fast and cheap? It won't be that good,

Fast and good? Sure, but it ain't cheap!

Good and cheap? Ok, but you'll have to wait a while.

Of course there are versions in between. In fact, I'm trying to decide what my own BodyBack programme is! It's not expensive compared to some, but neither could I justify the ridiculously low price I launched at last year – the results people get are just too good.

It's also not a 'drop a stone in a fortnight' programme, (average seems to be about 6–10lb in the first month), but then the weight stays off once it's off.

Have you ever tried the free/cheap option of something, only to discover it doesn't work?

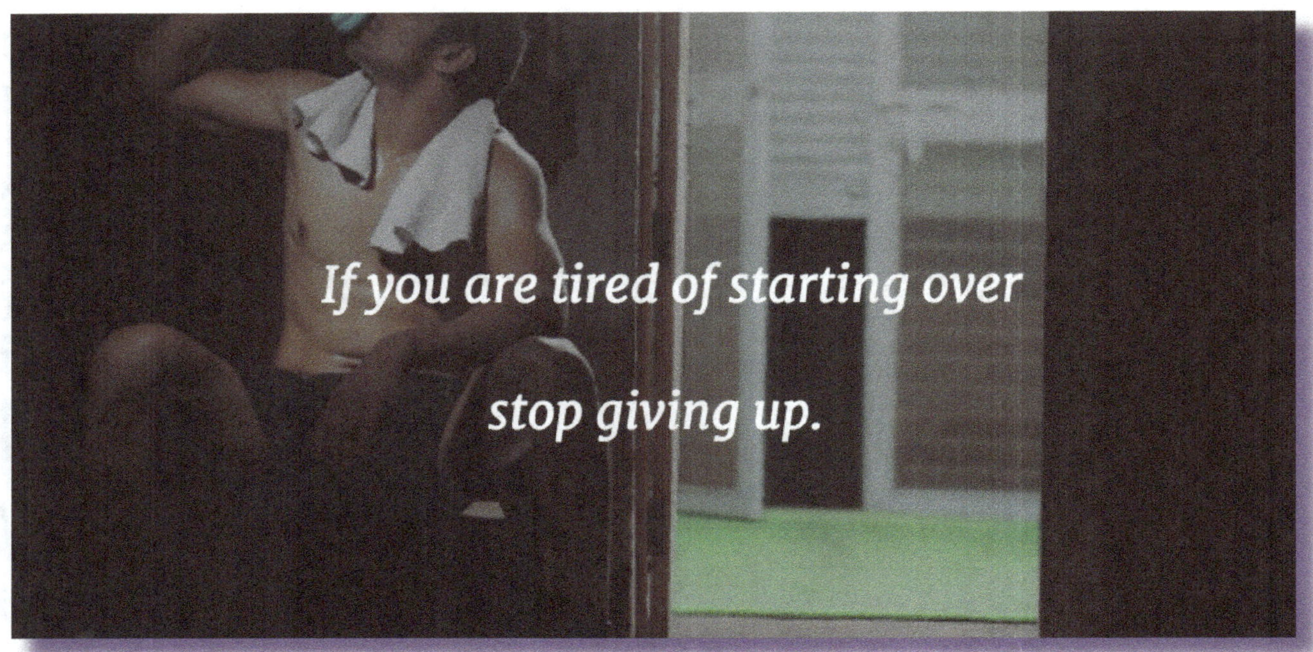

If you are tired of starting over, stop giving up. Simple really isn't it? If you can't seem to stop giving up, maybe you keep starting the wrong things.

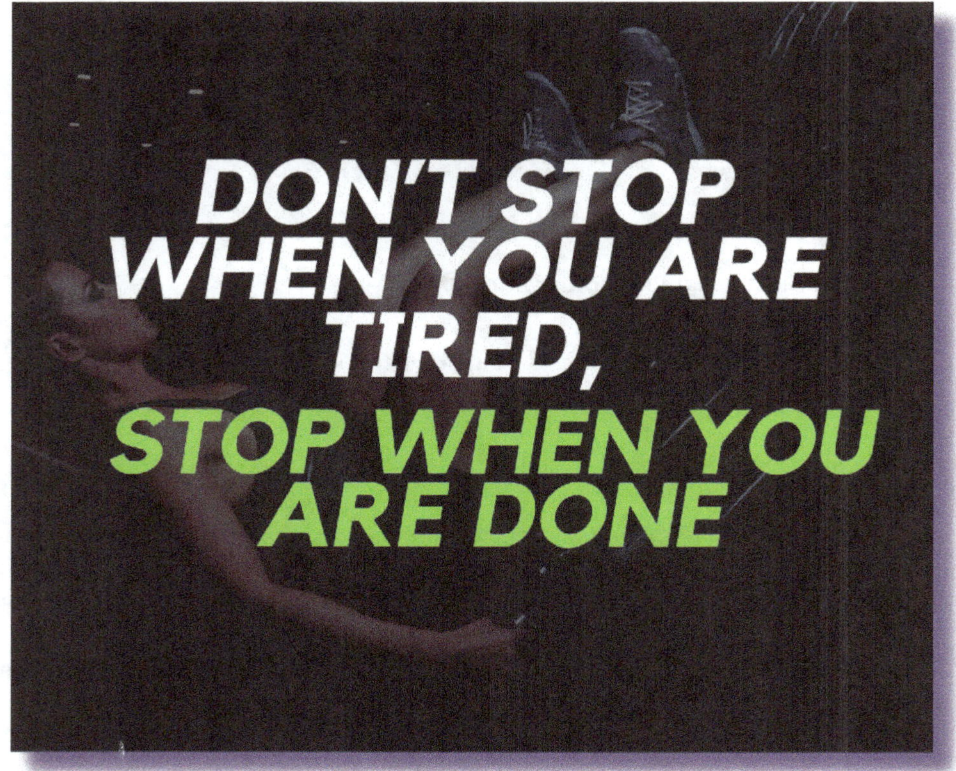

I don't mean put yourself in pain or make life utterly miserable, but you have to get out of your comfort zone to make progress.

In exercise this means feeling the 'ache' or 'burn' so that your muscles get stronger and more toned.

In life, I find most things worth having are worth putting effort into getting.

"DO IT ANYWAY, MOTIVATED OR NOT."

It is not effective to try and motivate yourself all of the time. You will NOT be motivated all of the time. It's very rare.

The trick, for want of a better word, is to get into the habit of doing it anyway, whether you feel motivated or not.

Nike use the phrase 'just do it' because they understand this.

When you try and give your kids a medicine they don't like the taste of, you tell them, just hold your nose and down it, 'just do it'.

So, that workout; that chopping vegetables; that buying fruit and putting it in your workbag/having it on your desk ... just do it.

> "There is nothing outside yourself that can ever enable you to get better, stronger, richer, quicker, or smarter. Everything is within. Everything exists. Seek nothing outside of yourself ."
>
> Miyamoto Musashi

Ponder on that for a bit.

Pretty empowering isn't it?

We want someone to save us, give us the answers, the permission.

We look far and wide for the solutions to our problems.

Turns out it was within our power all along.

It might be small (at the moment), it might be quiet.

But it's there. You just gotta dig it out.

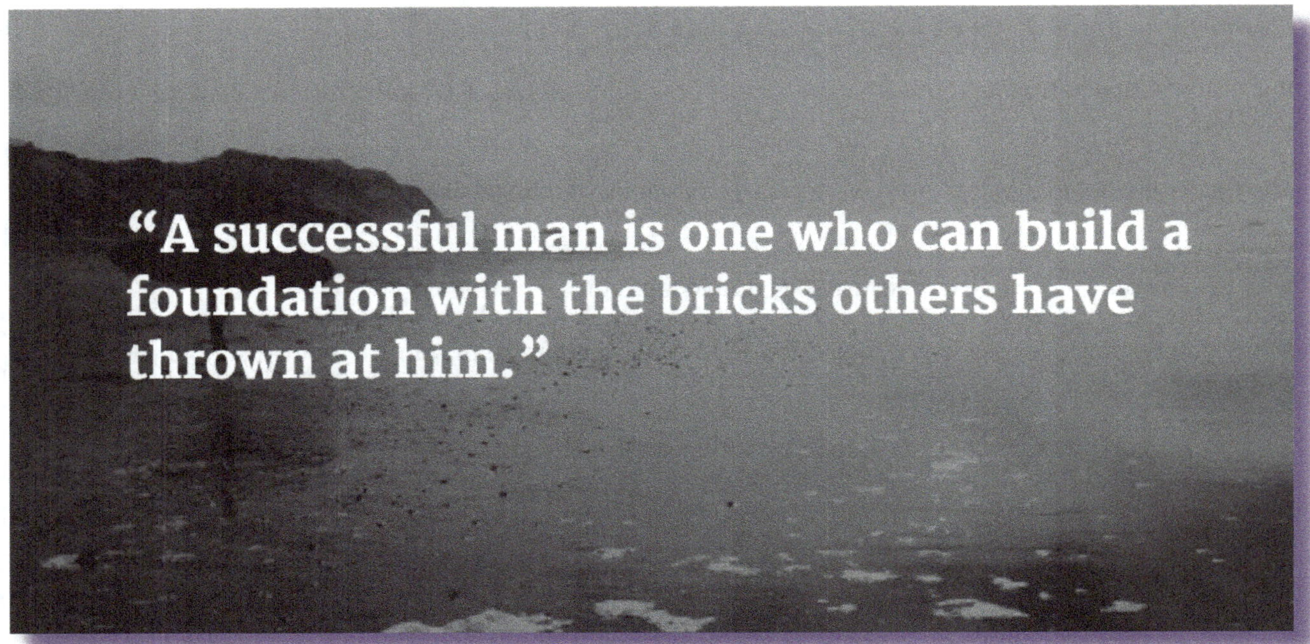

Turn a challenge into an opportunity. Turn obstacles into ladders. Make triumph out of adversity.

And, most magic of all, turn hate into love.

"COMMITMENT IS MORE THAN DECLARATION."

There's a difference between someone who really wants to reach their goals ...

... and someone who is 100% committed to taking the necessary steps to get there.

Tip? Write it down. Clearly and precisely.

Then SIGN IT. And date it.

Then show people, tell people, and put it somewhere you can't miss it (fridge door, perhaps?).

What are you committing to?

"YOU HAVE MORE POWER THAN YOU REALISE."

The only person you are destined to become is the person you decide to be. You have way more control over your future and even your current state than you probably know or believe.

Not believing this statement actually has a name, Learnt Helplessness.

Luckily, it can be unlearnt!

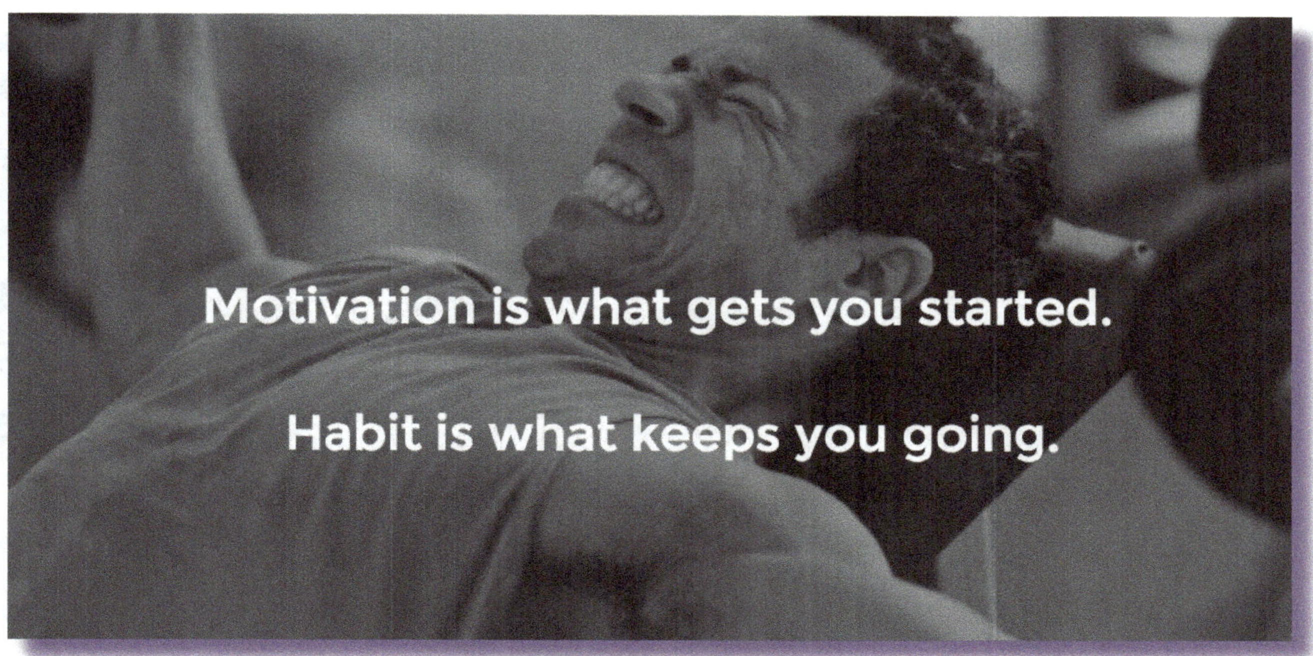

What does being on holiday/out of routine do to your food and exercise habits?

If your 'non-negotiable' habits are simple but prioritised enough, they should be able to slip into your day even though your usual routine is disrupted.

- 3 x weekly workout? Check

- lots of vegetables and protein with each meal? Check

- walking or general 'moving'? Probably not as much for me without the school run, but we'll walk to the shops and do some pre-winter gardening.

Have you planned your half-term week to include these non-negotiable habits?

"YOU HAD THE POWER ALL LONG, MY DEAR."
GLINDA, THE GOOD WITCH, WIZARD OF OZ.

It's true, and as Dorothy demonstrates, you don't even have to be a witch to find what you were looking for.

Sometimes you have to look inside instead of chasing rainbows.

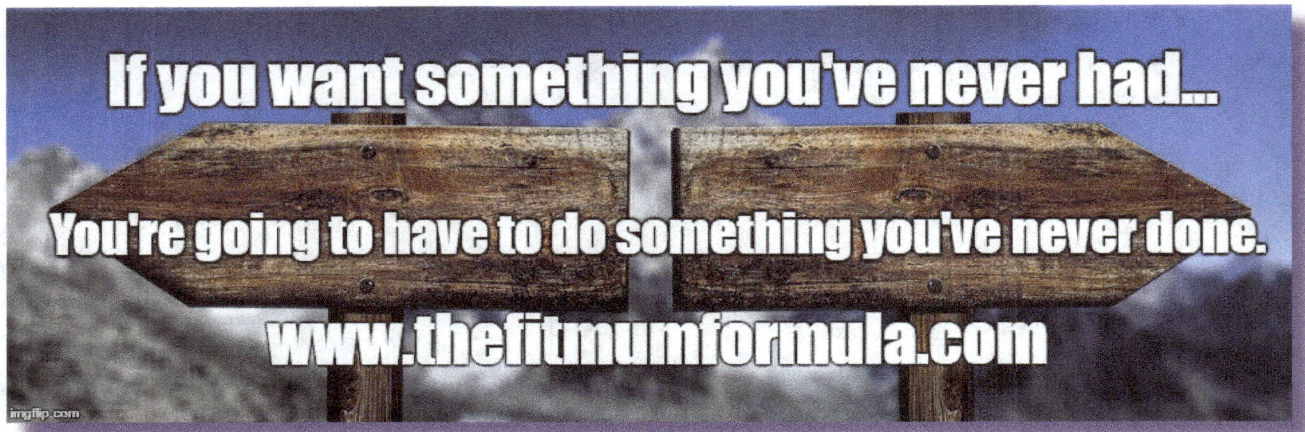

I think this is pretty much common sense ...

... but not commonly followed through.

Want change? Then change.

Not sure what to change?

Pick one thing, change that, give it enough time, assess results/change, tweak as necessary.

Not sure what to pick first? Pick anything! Or feel free to get in touch and I'll help you choose one simple thing you can change today.

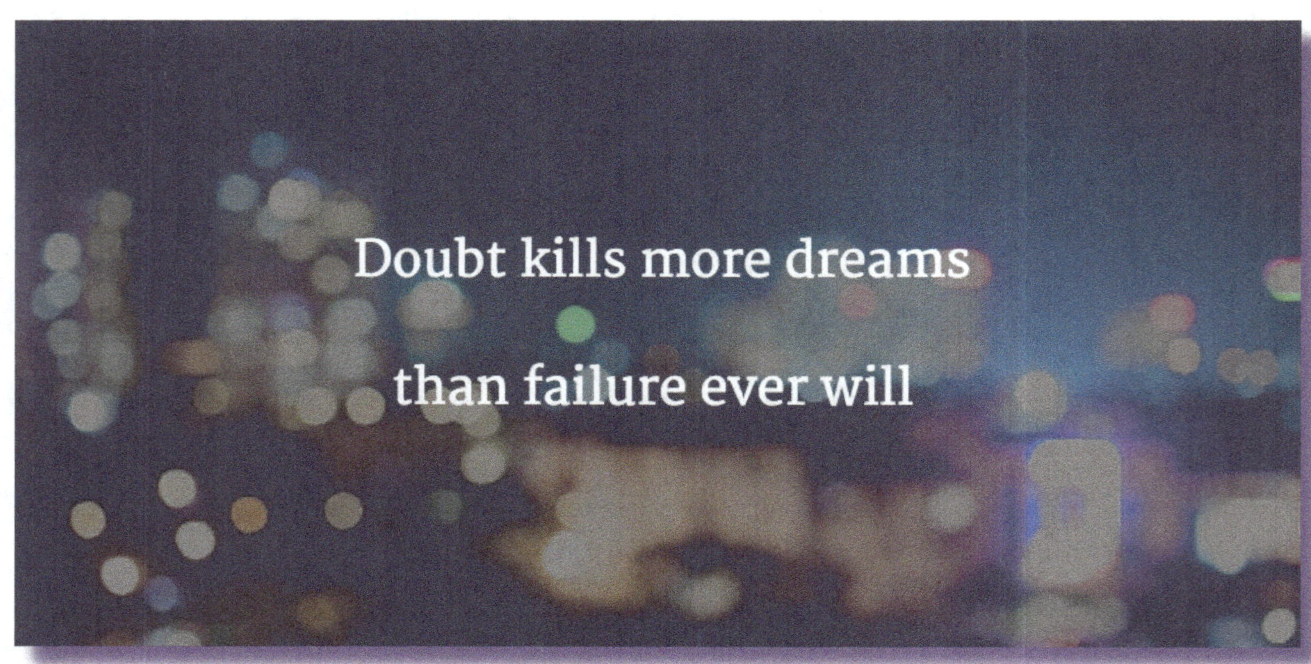

To reach your dreams you have to get over the doubt in your ability to reach them.

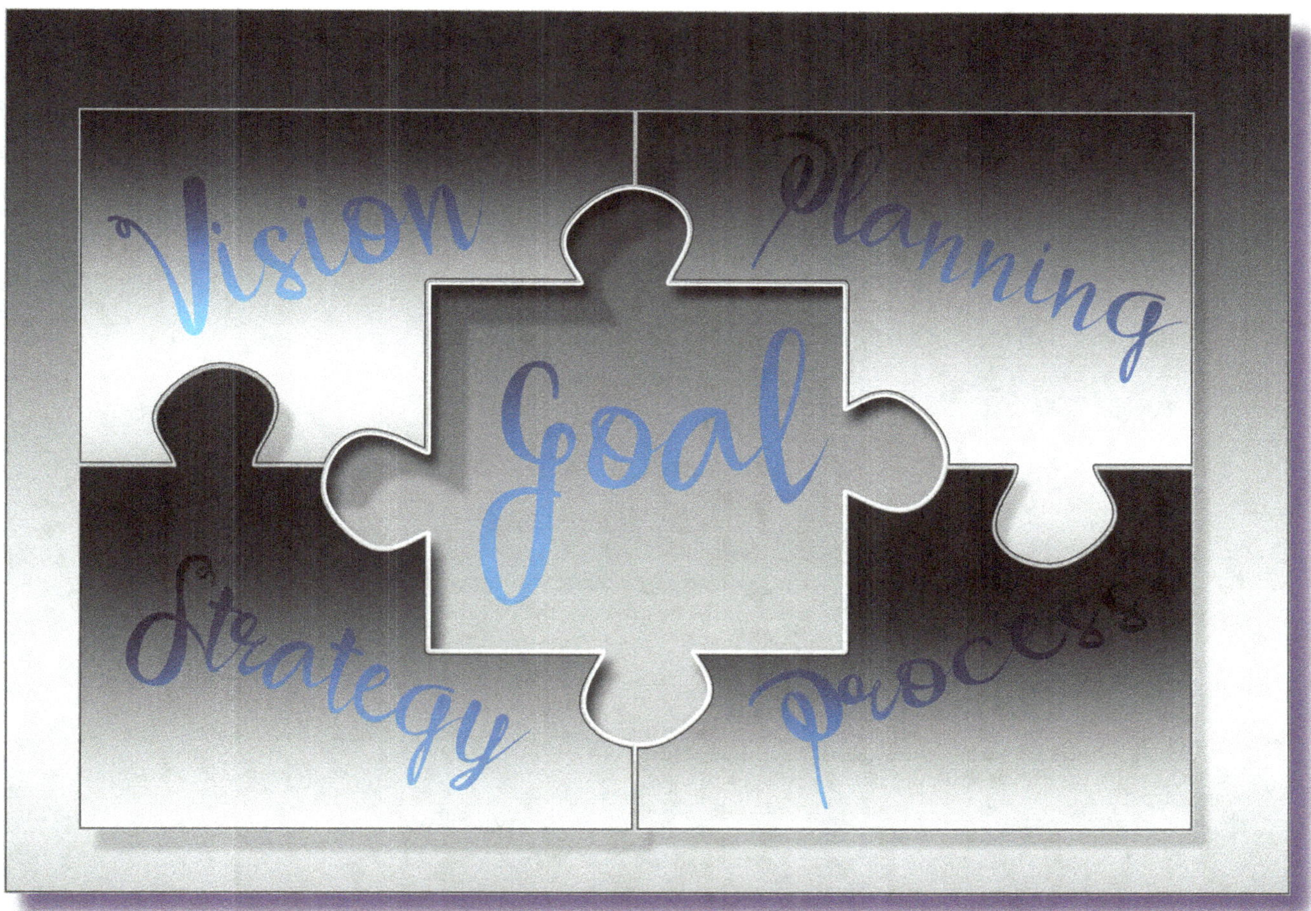

Outcome goals vs process goals.

Most people have an outcome goal; they want to lose x pounds, get into x size, run an x mile race.

While those can work, reaching set goals is not linear. It's rocky, challenging, and sometimes two steps forward, one (or two!) steps back, which means if you don't reach your set goal fast enough, or have a day when you seem to go backwards, it can be extremely disheartening.

And once you reach that set goal, then what?

If, on the other hand, your goal is to carry out the processes that ultimately get you to your goal, then this instils habits that you do consistently, always, trusting and having faith that the end result WILL come with persistence (and it will).

Eat the right food.

Do the workouts.

Walk.

Sleep.

Repeat indefinitely.

The results will come in time, and better than that they'll keep coming, and keep getting better .... so long as you're being consistent and persistent in the process.

DO SOMETHING TODAY THAT YOUR FUTURE SELF WILL THANK YOU FOR

You might not want to do that workout right now. You might prefer to drive in a warm car rather than put a coat on and walk. You might be too tired to do anything but eat biscuits and toast.

But in the next few hours, days, weeks and months, you will feel the effects of your choices.

Will your body be thanking you for the benefits of your actions, or resenting impulsive choices?

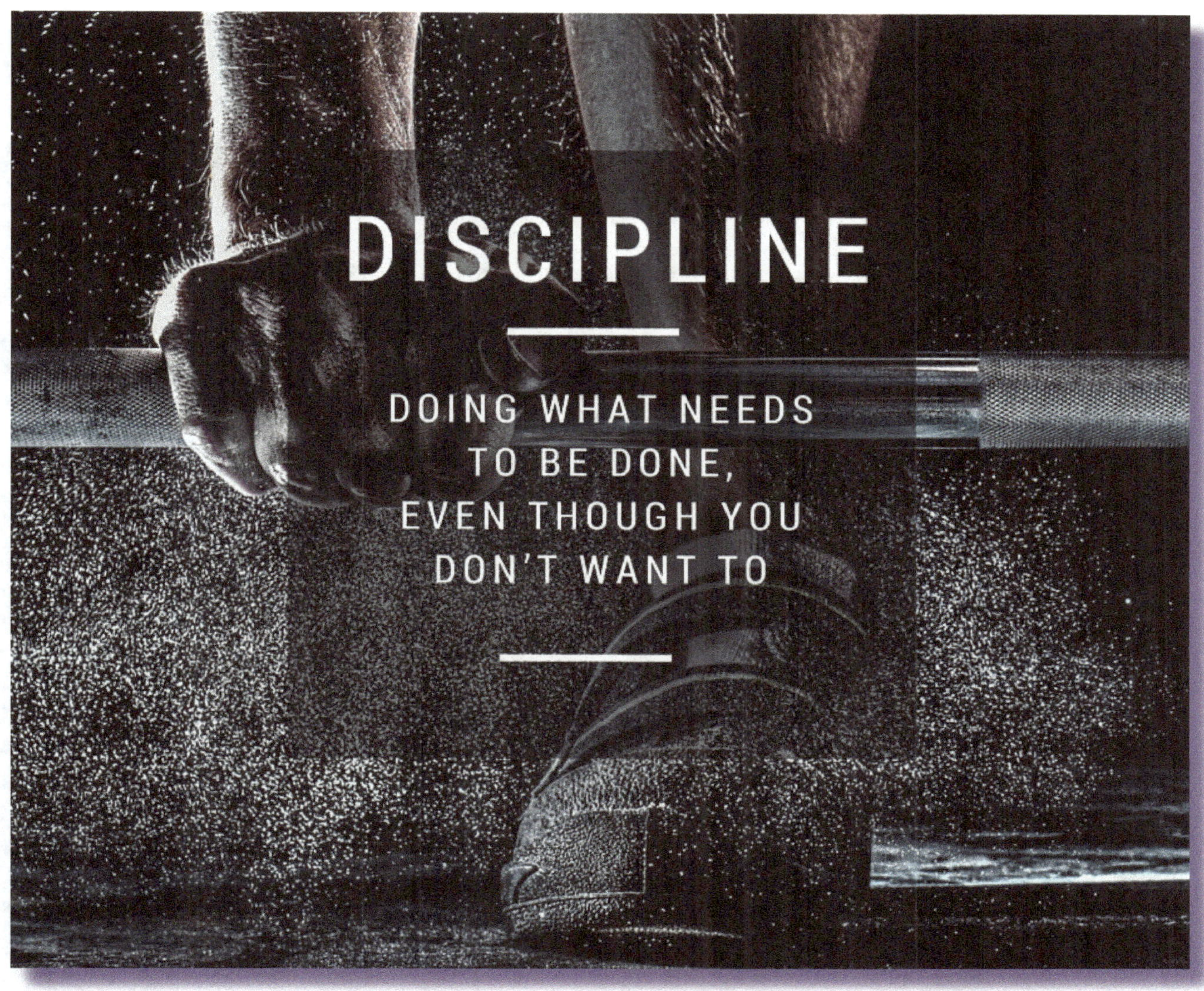

You won't always feel like working out. You won't always feel like making a healthy meal. But if you think about it, you don't always feel like having a shower, doing the school run, or going to work either.

Yet you do it, because these things have become not just habits, but you have decided consciously that they are important enough to do them anyway.

How important are your body, your health, your energy levels and self-confidence to you?

Are they worth 'doing things anyway' for?

Tip: it probably will feel like a 'no' before you do them. Once done, you'll realise they were completely worth the effort.

Give it a try.

> # When you want to succeed as bad as you want to breath, then you'll be successful

Maybe you just don't want it bad enough. That's OK. Don't waste your time and energy going after things you don't even want.

If you do really want something? Think beyond that. Why do you want it? On a scale of one to ten how badly do you want it? How would you feel when you got it? What would your life look like when you got it?

Good? Better?

Then go after it.

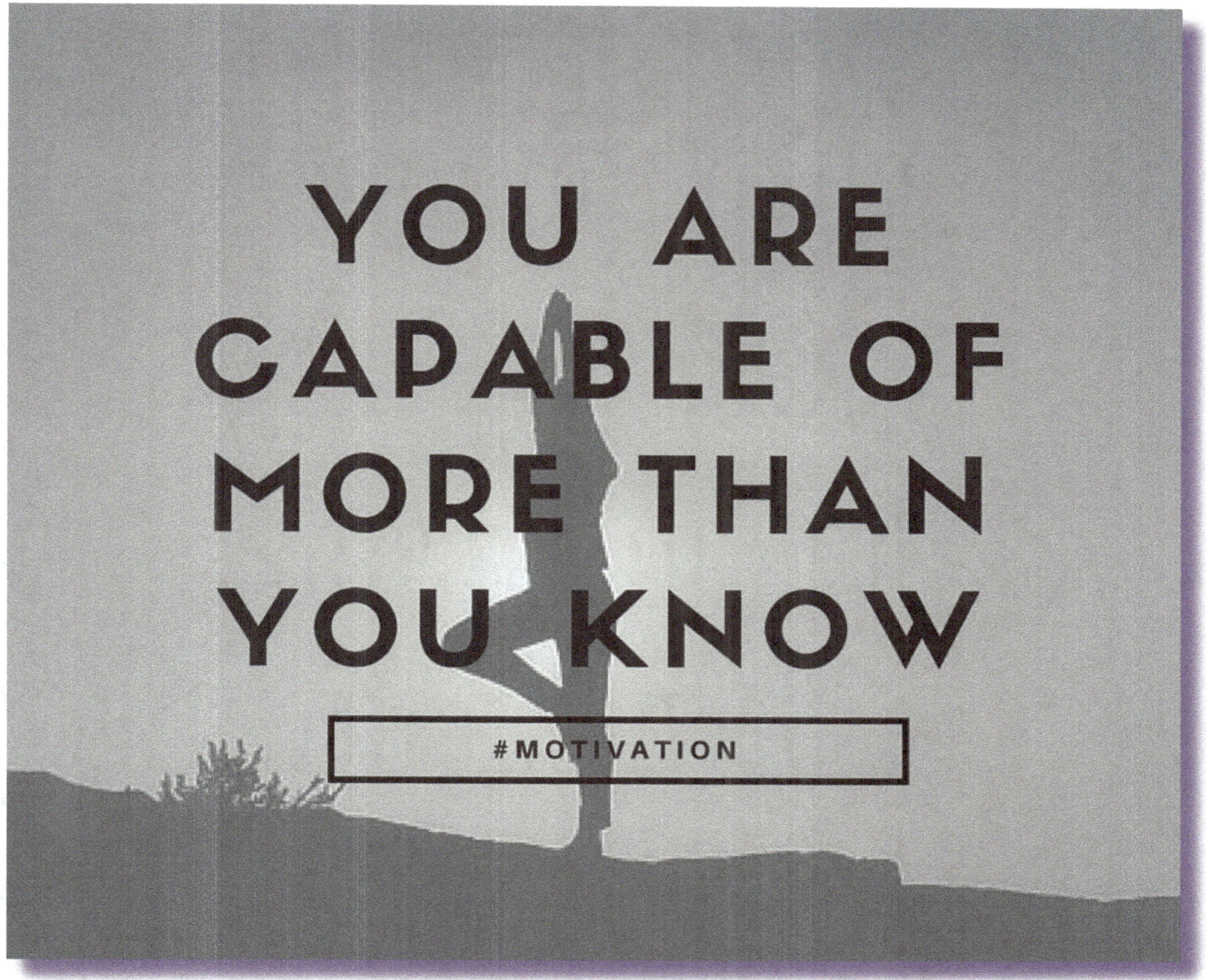

Self-efficacy is the belief in yourself than you can accomplish something.

If you don't believe you can achieve something, why would you bother trying it?

The best way to get this confidence and self-efficacy is by seeing the results for yourself.

Can you really know for sure you can't do it if you haven't tried? No, you can't know for sure.

Failed last time? That was then. You are a new, older, wiser person since then, even if it's only a week!

You are different, which means what you can achieve will be more/different.

Don't believe me? Try it anyway.

If it doesn't work out? Look at why.

Maybe your heart isn't in it after all. Maybe it's the wrong 'thing' (diet, job, exercise) for you. You can get guidance on finding the 'best' things for you, but even when people come to me for help, two of the first questions I ask are 'what's worked for you in the past' and 'what hasn't worked for you'. Then we have something to start with, to go on. But you won't know the answers to these questions if you haven't tried.

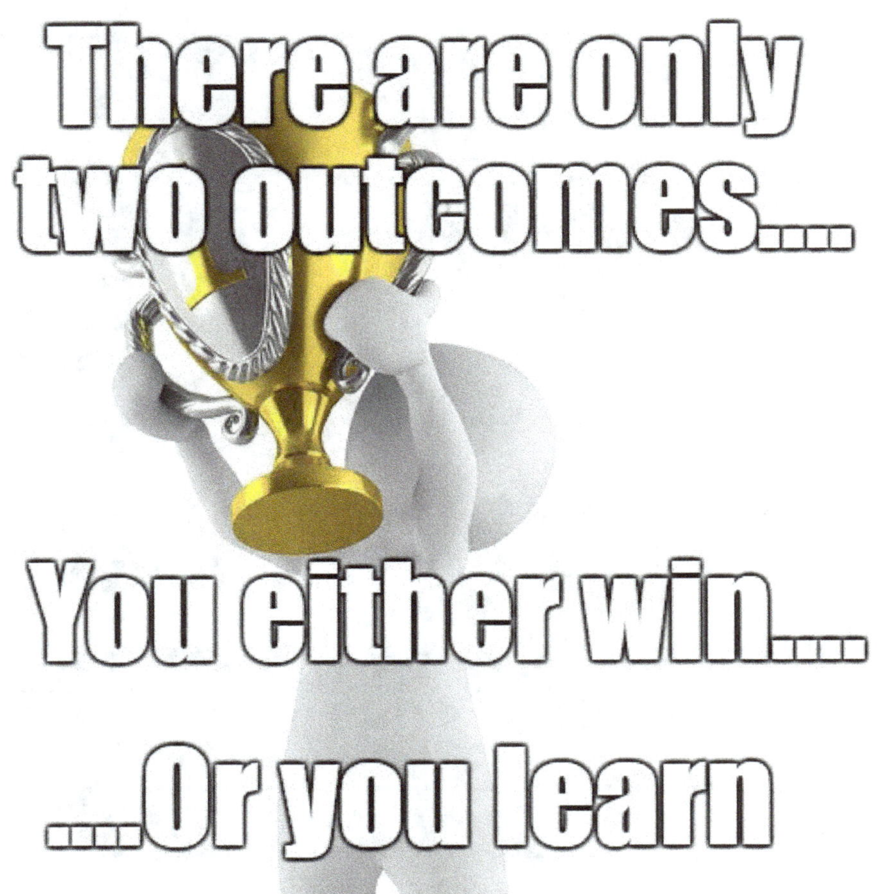

Our brain learns new skills by failing. Through trial and error, you eventually land on something that works.

Mastery happens by letting go of what hasn't worked, refining what has, and repeating what works over and over, until you become a master of it.

But hardly anyone gets it right first time. There will always be errors and lessons along the way.

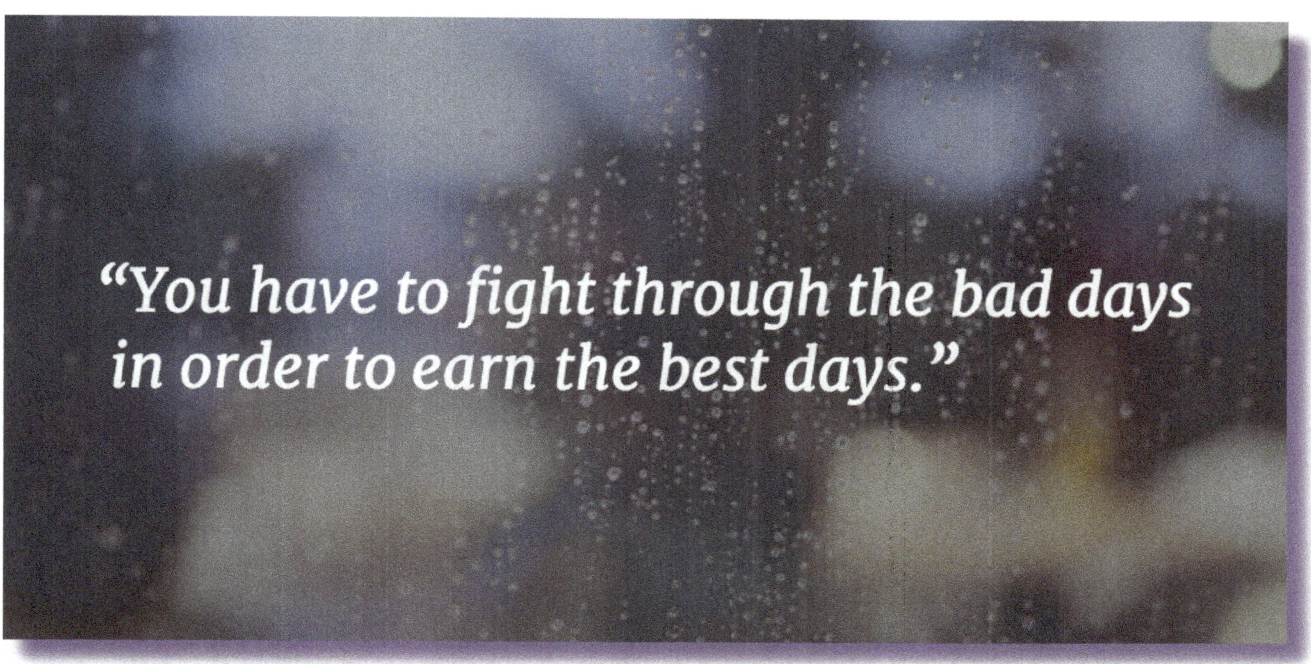

Everything worth having is worth fighting for. Nobody ever got anything worth having without trying.

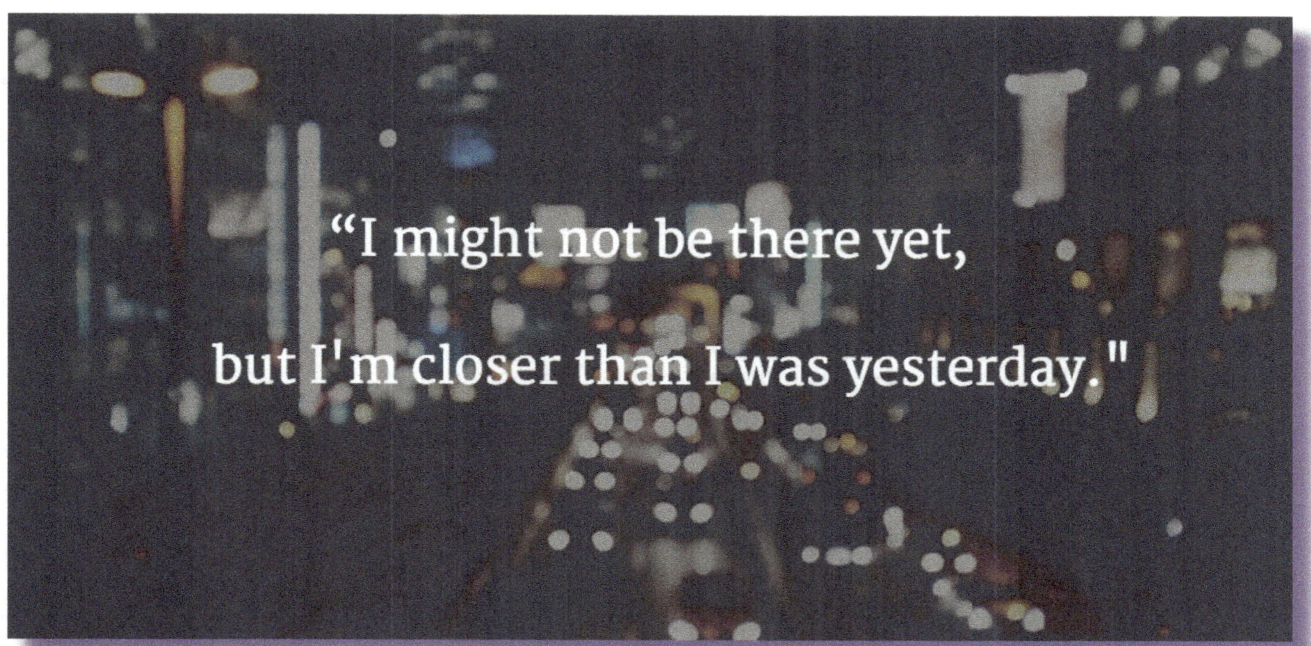

It doesn't matter where you come from. It doesn't matter how fast you go. As long as you're going in the right direction.

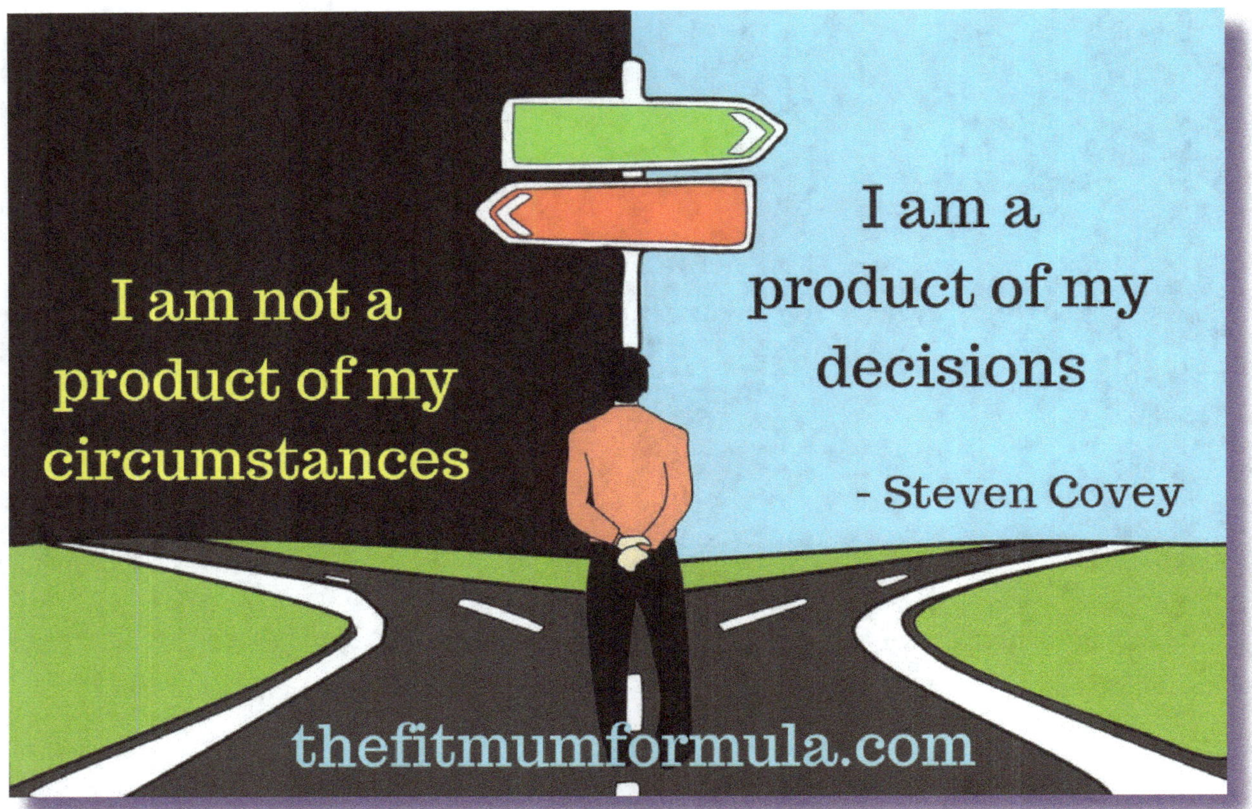

There is a choice in every circumstance. Not always an easy one.

Sometimes you're stuck between a rock and a hard place.

Usually something will have to be sacrificed to get something else.

Want to work out early morning as you don't have time during the day?

Then yes, you'll have to get up earlier.

Everyone tucking into sticky toffee pudding but you're trying to lose weight? You'll need to serve yourself a smaller portion than them.

All the Christmas chocolates and pies on special offer? They're even cheaper if you don't buy any ;)

The shops might tell you 'buy now or pay more later', but they've neglected to give you that third option – don't buy!

Change the story from "I should", "I could", "I might", "I can't"

to "I CHOOSE TO".

It's way more powerful.

REWIRING YOUR BRAIN FOR SUCCESS.

It is your SUBCONSCIOUS mind that determines most of your actions.

I want to give you an excerpt from Christine Hassler's book *Expectation Hangover*:

"Let's start with some basic neuroscience. Repetitive thoughts form what are called neural nets in our brains, which are clusters of chemically connected or functionally associated neurons. What that means is that if you think the same thought or type of thought over and over, it forms an actual physical cluster of neurons in your brain. Over time the neural nets create 'grooves' in the brain that your thoughts gravitate toward. For instance, if you repeatedly think, 'I'm not good enough,' you create a neural net around that limited pattern of thought. Once the neural net is formed, it becomes habitual to think in the direction of 'I'm not good enough.' Thus you will tend to see things that occur in your life through the lens of 'I'm not good enough.' Since repeated patterns of neural activity change neural structure, you can use your mind to change your brain. This is called self-directed neuroplasticity. Bottom line: neurons that fire together, wire together. You can learn to stimulate different parts of your brain, which will improve your wellbeing and functioning."

If you tell yourself repeatedly that you "can't resist x food" or you "just can't get motivated to exercise", that conscious message gets ingrained into your subconscious mind.

Can you see how this leads to destructive behaviours?

Change the messages you tell yourself each day and, if done repeatedly, they will become subconscious, and in turn translate into actions.

YOU ARE A BITCH!

Let's imagine a friend of yours, or a close acquaintance, we'll call her Jennifer.

Jennifer needs to lose some weight. You know it, she knows it. But she's struggling. She can't stick to her plan, always falls off the wagon, can't seem to get organised to find time to exercise. So this is what you tell her:

"You are just making excuses. Jennifer you are fat and lazy and you probably always will be at this rate. You never stick to anything, you have no willpower, and you are completely incapable – you will never succeed at this. You've always failed in the past, why should now be any different? There is no evidence to suggest that you will ever be able to lose weight, you just don't have it in you. Why are you even bothering to try? It's just not going to be worth the effort, I wouldn't bother if I were you."

What an absolute cow! Can you honestly say you would talk to someone else like this? I sincerely hope not. But you do. Every day, you and so many other women talk to themselves like this every day.

Change the self-talk, will you? Depreciation was never an effective method of motivation. Instead, put yourself (or Jennifer, if it's easy to picture someone else for now) on a pedestal.

Tell her that she is important. She is worth the effort. She *can* do this. Tell her she might need some help and support. She might need to learn some new skills and have help figuring out where she's been going wrong.

But she absolutely *will* succeed and she is absolutely *is* worth it.

Now go and find a pedestal and sit on it.

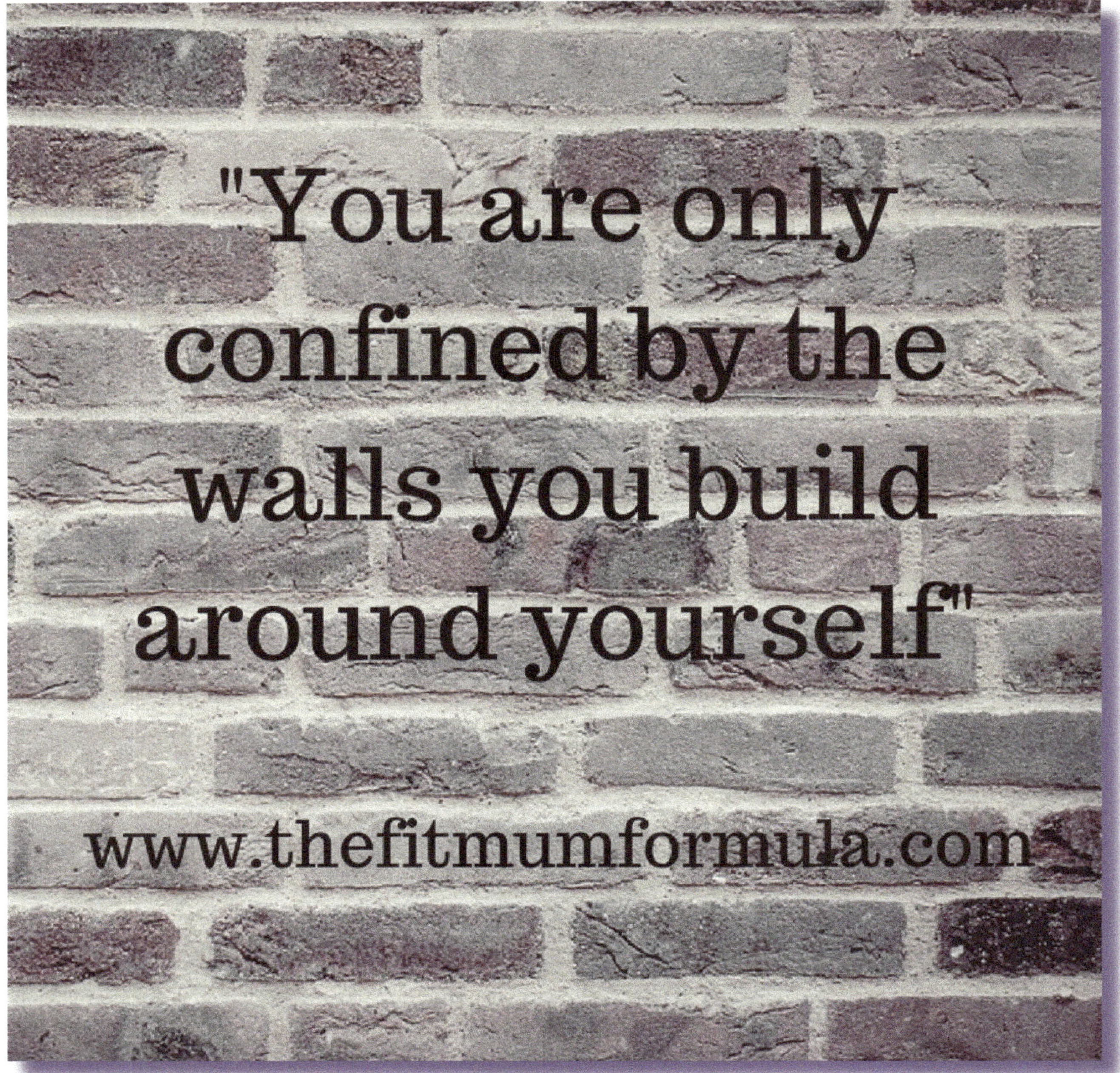

Are you making life hard for yourself?

Did you put yourself in a pigeon hole?

Maybe you've always been overweight, so perhaps that's 'just your metabolism'?

Perhaps you continually self-sabotage and buy all the Christmas chocolate on offer, even though you know you won't be able to 'pace yourself' at home.

And here's the most common limit I see – excuses. Maybe you genuinely don't have time to do a one-hour workout; perhaps you could commit to 10 body weight squats every time the kettle boils (that would be quite often in my house, I like tea!)

Stop placing boundaries around what you can accomplish and the possibilities open up.

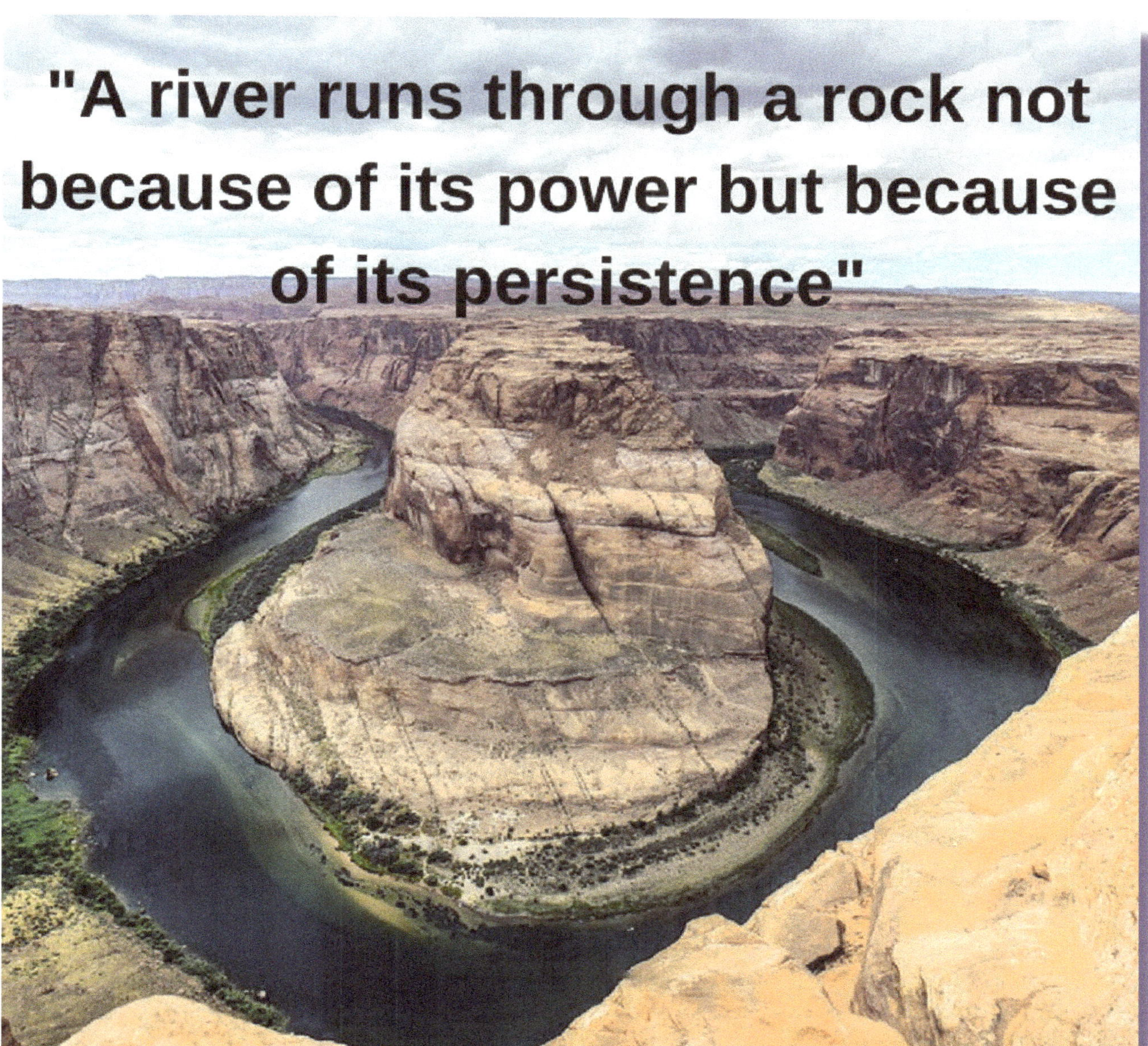

Many people jump head first into a diet and exercise plan, making huge changes and attempting to do everything all at once. This rarely works. It's unlikely to be sustainable.

What does work is consistency and persistence.

Lots of veg. Lots of walking. Enough protein. Limiting but not excluding treats. Some muscle-building activity a few times a week. Good sleep. Little stress. Doing things that make you happy.

Repeat, repeat, repeat.

FINAL THOUGHTS

Now the feminist-anti-discrimination-non-judgemental-love-yourself crew are going to batter me for the rest of this book since I seem to be implying that you should make an effort and not 'let yourself go'.

And they are right.

You are not your body.

You are not your skin (wrinkly, spotty, or otherwise).

You are not your age.

You are a human with a soul and a personality and you are special just as you are for being you. And that makes you extremely valuable.

YOU are a very important person.

Not convinced?

Ask your kids. Ask your partner. Ask your parents, your best friend, your brothers and sisters.

Everybody loves you and wants you to be healthy and happy, confident and contented.

If your relationship with food, with your body, and the way you treat and prioritise your physical self (or rather, don't prioritise it) is stopping you from being all these things, then that needs to change.

I want to help you do that. My door will never be shut to the people who need my help.

FIX IT

HOW TO PERSONALISE YOUR DIET PLAN

There is no such thing as the perfect diet plan. Sorry about that. Or let me rephrase that. There is such thing an almost perfect diet plan, for a particular person, on a particular day, but since we can only know so much about that person on any given day, it makes it near impossible to make a diet plan that's perfect for two different people, or even for the same person but on different days!

That being said, if you know how to tweak your diet according to a few key circumstances, you will be adapting what you eat to what your body needs, and that's the secret to getting it right, whatever your goals.

Establishing your goals

The first thing you have to do is work out exactly what it is you want to achieve. Is it to pack on 15 lb of muscle and compete in a power lift meeting? Is it to address digestive problems like IBS and to stop needing an hour's afternoon nap and 10 coffees a day just to get through? Did you splurge a little over Christmas and want to lose that half a stone?

Each goal will have a unique starting point. For example, to gain muscle you'll need to eat many more calories and combine this with weightlifting; to solve digestive issues you might try eliminating one suspect food at a time and see if you're reacting to something. To keep it simple **I'm going to address the most common goal people come to me for, weight loss.**

The solution to weight loss is simple, but not easy. It's simple because all you have to do is eat fewer calories than you burn. Unfortunately, hunger and cravings tend to go up when we do this, and energy levels can go down, along with our willpower and ability to stick to the diet. Ultimately, the best diet is the one you can stick to, but it has to fit the following criteria:

- keeps you feeling full

- stops you craving unhelpful foods

- leaves you with plenty of energy

- fits into your life (work, being a parent, etc.)

- gets results (in this case weight loss)

What is required to do this varies from person to person. Some people may need more fibre and protein, more or fewer starchy carbohydrates or fat, or can go for longer or shorter periods between eating.

Pay attention to your hunger, food cravings, energy levels and mood, as well as weight loss and measurements. Write them alongside a food diary so you can see what affects you in different ways. This will help you decide if you need to make changes anywhere to help you continue and make progress. At the end of this chapter you'll find some diary templates for you to print out or photocopy and fill in.

How you adjust your plan depends on how you are feeling (hunger, energy and cravings) and how your body is responding (fat or weight, loss or gain). How you feel can change from day to day, so it really pays to stop and ask yourself how you're feeling and let your diet adapt accordingly.

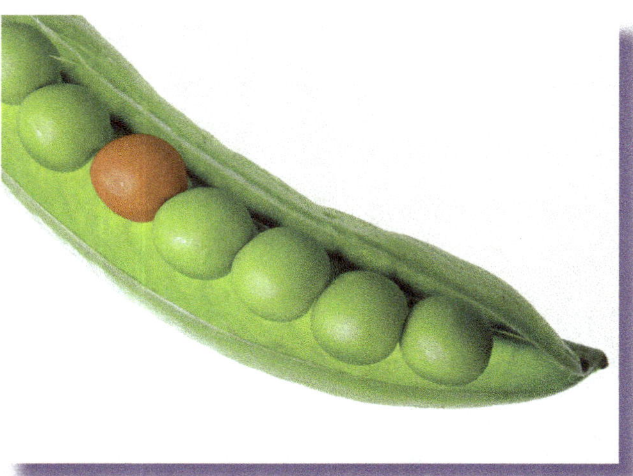

HUNGER, CRAVINGS, ENERGY, FAT BURNING, MOOD

The wonderful thing about The Fit Mum Formula's methods is that they are adaptable, so that you make it fit YOUR body and YOUR lifestyle, since we believe we are all different, no one strict plan will suit everyone. The meal guidelines in the Food chapter are a great starting point, then you can adjust it depending on how you respond.

How you adjust your plan depends on how you are feeling (hunger, energy and cravings) and how your body is responding (fat or weight loss or gain).

Using these as keys, you can tweak what you eat and do until you reach an optimum method that works for you, one where you are not hungry, don't have cravings, have tonnes of energy and are sleeping well, and of course you are losing fat and toning up!

Side effects

Something you need to be aware of when starting the programme is, as with anything new, if you are not used to eating and exercising this way then you may experience some side effects while your body adjusts and, most importantly, switches from burning sugar as fuel (or muscle turned into sugar) to burning fat. It varies how long this takes but is usually between 3–14 days for most people, during which you may experience headaches, low energy, harder workouts, quicker muscle fatigue, food cravings, difficulty sleeping, dips in mood and changes in bowel habits. These are perfectly normal and do not mean that the plan is not working or that it is not for you, just that you need to allow your body time to respond appropriately. There's even a name for this phenomenon, 'carb flu'!

Some things you can do to ease yourself through this stage are:

- **eat plenty of protein and fibre** (low starch vegetables, salad and low sugar fruits); increasing consumption of these should be your first step

- **slightly increase your intake of carbohydrates** at first; you can lower them when your body has had time to adjust

- **pre-emptive eating**; eat before you get too hungry, so that you prevent the release of too many stress hormones to raise blood sugar, and to prevent you from overcompensating later and ultimately eating more overall

- **use cocoa powder** (1–2 tbsp. in hot water, sweetened with stevia if you like) to curb cravings, and green tea for energy

- **BCAA**'s (Branch Chain Amino Acids), and Fibre (psyllium husks) in supplement forms can help you through energy dips and hunger

- use **GABA-inducing** (a relaxing neurotransmitter in your body) **herbs** such as **chamomile** and **lemon balm** tea to reduce stress levels, in addition to lots of walking

- **don't be tempted to go fat free**; natural fats in meat, dairy, fish, nuts, avocado, coconuts, etc. will slow digestion and keep you feeling satisfied

Eat often

I advise regular eating – 3 meals plus 3 snacks a day – until your body is more able to draw on fat stores for energy. Skipping meals when your body is not good at reaching for fat stores in the 'starvation' situation will leave you tired, hungry and irritable, or 'hangry'! Getting hungry will also mean you reach for sugary, fatty, starchy foods, which are counterproductive when it comes to fat burning. In time you may notice you don't need as many snacks, as your metabolism gets 'food' from your fat stores when it needs to; this is an excellent sign!

Hunger, cravings, energy, fat burning, mood

These three things are what will determine your success on the programme. If you are too hungry, have strong cravings or have low energy then, unless you have a willpower of steel, you will eventually cave in to sweet, salty, fatty, carbohydrate rich foods to address these feelings. Ironically these are exactly the things that you should not eat.

The aim is to find your optimum diet and exercise programme that keeps hunger and cravings low, and energy levels high, and what is required to do this varies from person to person. The programme I have set out will suit many people as it is, but it is a middle-ground version. Some people may need more fibre and protein, more or fewer starchy carbohydrates or fat, or can go for longer or shorter periods between eating.

Pay attention to your hunger, food cravings, energy levels and mood. Write them alongside your food diary, or fill in all the forms below, so you can see what affects you in different ways. This will help you decide if you need to make changes anywhere to help you continue and make progress.

HUNGER

- **fibre** provides bulk and also slows digestion; eat lots of vegetables, salad, and fruit rather than starch to get your fibre; fibre supplements (such as psyllium husks), taken with or between meals, can also help when hunger is a big issue

- **protein** is much more satiating than carbohydrates and takes longer to digest; protein powder provides a healthy protein fix between meals, or when you just need something quickly

- **fat** does not make you fat (excess calories, combined with a body which likes to store calories rather than burn them, does that), but it is quite satiating, and essential to body functioning; choose full-fat products if you like, just skip the (not so satiating) starch

- **vinegar** slows down digestion so food stays in your stomach for longer and decreases the amount of insulin released after eating; any type of vinegar will do; use it instead of, or as an ingredient in, salad dressings

CRAVINGS

- **cocoa** decreases cravings for sweet and starchy foods by stimulating the pleasure seekers dopamine and serotonin in the brain

- **fibre** can help control cravings by sending messages to our brain that we are full, and therefore that we need no more food

- **xylitol** is a natural, yet low calorie, sweetener that provides a sweet hit, while at the same time encouraging a feeling of fullness, so two benefits in one

- **protein powder**, cravings can sometimes be the result of a lack of certain amino acids, so adequate protein intake can help this; branch chain amino acids (BCAA's) can be taken as a supplement, however, it is always better to get amino acids and protein from food or quality protein shakes between meals if possible

ENERGY

- **cocoa** provides sustained energy and many other benefits; enjoy 1–3 cups of cocoa a day if or when you need it

- **coffee** should be restricted to no more than 3 cups of good quality fresh coffee, ideally in the morning; do not use coffee as a substitute for proper eating, and if you feel it is impacting negatively on cravings and hunger then go without it

- **green tea** has less caffeine than black tea, and also contains theanine, which relaxes the mind, so you stay focused and alert, but calm rather than wired

- **BCAA**'s in supplement form help some people maintain energy levels, and are often taken first thing in the morning if you like to work out before eating

- **black tea**, like green, contains caffeine (slightly more than green tea) and theanine, contributing to a calm but focused disposition

- **herbal tea**'s containing energising ginseng and ginger can energise without caffeine

FAT BURNING

- **green tea** reduces the body's reaction to stress, thereby reducing fat storage; it also stimulates fat burning at a genetic level and in the liver

- **omega-3** fats, either as a supplement or in fish oils or flax, despite being fats themselves, actually stimulate the body into burning fat

- **warming spices**, known as thermogenic spices, such as cinnamon, ginger, chilli and cayenne, can speed up the metabolism, aid digestion, slightly encourage fat burning, and (some studies show) also reduce the amount of calories eaten in the meal

- **cocoa** stabilises blood sugar, thereby discouraging fat storage

MOOD

- **omega-3** fats, either as a supplement or in fish oils or flax, have been shown to be so effective at regulating brain activity (including concentration, mood, and psychiatric disorders) that it is sometimes used as a first port of call instead of medication when treating conditions naturally (of course, if you think you have any of the above conditions please see your GP first)

- **cocoa** enhances serotonin and dopamine levels, which are powerful mood enhancers; it also stabilises blood sugar, which in turn stabilises concentration and mood

- **tryptophan**, an amino acid that makes 5-HTP, encourages serotonin production, leading to improvements in mood, sleep, anxiety levels and cognitive functioning; tryptophan is found in poultry, shellfish, sea vegetables such as seaweed, leafy greens like spinach, and sunflower seeds; it is available in supplement form.

- **herbs** that promote relaxation and stress relief, such as valerian, chamomile, hops, lemon balm and passion flower, can be taken as supplements, tea infusions and tinctures

N.B. Please seek advice from a registered naturopath regarding doses if planning on taking any supplements, and inform them of any conditions you have or medication taken.

Progress troubleshooting

WEIGHT

This is actually a poor indication of your progress since muscle weighs a lot more than fat, so a slim but tight and lean person might actually weigh a lot more than a larger, flabbier person. Of course, if you have a lot of weight to lose then you will lose weight if you are following the programme correctly. By all means weigh yourself if you have a lot of weight to lose, but don't use this as the only indicator of progress (and do it first thing in the morning only, food and drink consumed will sway results; and only once a week, in minimal clothing). It can actually be more helpful where fat loss has not occurred (see below), as it could indicate whether you might be following a 'weight loss' programme instead, in other words you're losing water and muscle.

BODY FAT COMPOSITION

The percentage measurement of fat in comparison to 'everything else' (i.e. bone, organs, muscle and water). Optimum body fat percentages are 15%–25% for women and 8%–15% for men, and I rate Tanita body composition scales (although there are many good ones on the market). They vary in accuracy, so the important thing is to get on them while every other variable is constant: first thing in the morning before you eat and drink; wearing only underwear is ideal; and only do it once a week.

Note that at different times during a woman's menstrual cycle you will hold on to more or less water so look at the bigger picture over a couple of cycles, there may be fluctuations, but if you are losing fat this measurement should be going down overall. Due to the varying accuracy of body fat scales, rather than trusting your result as an absolute truth, use it as a marker to see if you are going up or down with each week. Notice the overall trend rather than getting fixated over the actual numbers.

I've written more about Body Fat Percentage here: http://thefitmumformula.com/blog/what-is-body-fat-percentage/

N.B. Carbohydrates hold on to water, so during the first week of reducing your starch consumption you may lose a significant amount of water. Since water is classed under 'everything else' on body composition scales, proportionately it will tell you your body fat % has gone up. This is not the case, and results will appear more consistent and accurate once this initial water loss phase has passed.

MEASUREMENTS

If you can do it accurately with a tape measure then this is better than weight alone. When someone is losing a lot of muscle as weight then they could have smaller measurements, but not always, since they could be gaining fat at the same time, which weighs less even though it takes up more space (it's less dense). But with muscle loss your body shape won't change as much in the way that it does with fat loss, as fat loss occurs in different and specific areas of the body (you'll look more defined).

Women may see fat loss on the waist, hip and thigh areas, while men see it primarily on the waist. Thighs may slim down, but overall hip measurement may not go down since it is largely bone and muscle (and strong gluteals are what give women pert bottoms!). Notice your skin and muscle tone. Are you smaller and flabbier (muscle loss), or smaller and tighter (fat loss)? Again, measure at the same time each week and under the same conditions.

HUNGER, FOOD CRAVINGS AND ENERGY LEVELS

You may or may not be losing fat and building muscle but, either way, battling hunger and cravings, and having low energy levels is unsustainable, as willpower is exhaustible and you will eventually give in or give up altogether. So having these three issues under control is vital, whatever progress you are making.

Keeping a record of how you are feeling can show you if things are improving, and point you in the direction of what you can do to make your new lifestyle sustainable and enjoyable, as well as effective for fat loss.

WHAT YOUR RESULTS SAY

The caveat to this guideline: you are special because you are you, there is no one else quite like you, and therefore you have to play detective and work out how to tweak your diet, exercise and lifestyle to match your body.

I would dearly love to write you a plan, say do this, stick to it and you'll get results fast, but I'd be lying because what works for one person will not be quite right for the next. But I am here to guide you through this process and help you test, tweak and assess until we find what makes you thrive at your very best.

You have gained weight

Have you also gained muscle (shown as a decrease in body fat %)? Muscle weighs more than fat, so building muscle (which will in turn burn fat since it is very 'metabolically active') will weigh more, and you still might be making progress. Gaining muscle while burning fat will make you smaller despite weighing more, so look at your measurements to see if you have changed size or shape.

If you have not lost fat, then you need to tweak your programme to suit your individual genetic make-up – perhaps you need more sleep, fewer or more fat or carbohydrates, fewer or even a few *more* calories can even get you shifting fat and get you over plateaus since your body will most likely compensate by revving up your metabolism!

If you are satisfying your hunger and cravings by reaching for the very foods you crave (most likely high in sugar, fat and starch, as this is what we are biologically programmed to crave for quick energy fixes when blood sugar gets too low) then you will almost certainly not lose fat and quite possibly gain it.

Keep a diet diary as you may not even be aware of what and how much you are eating throughout the day. Also, be aware of how stress may be increasing hunger and cravings while decreasing energy – not enough sleep or going too long between eating will almost certainly have this effect. If your weight gain is not a positive gain in muscle mass (and decrease in body fat) then try the following:

- follow the programme – lots of **lean protein and vegetables, and some fruit**

- **reduce starchy carbohydrate** intake *but don't cut it out completely!*

- **get enough fat** to feel satisfied and energised, not too much to increase calories excessively; do not follow a predominantly low fat diet

- use **pre-emptive eating**; eat before hunger sets in to prevent you from over-compensating later

- increase **exercise** (high intensity workouts and walking)

- check that **catalyst foods** (that make you want more and more of them) and stress are not making your hunger, energy and cravings worse

You have lost weight

Whether this is a good or a bad thing depends on whether the weight you have lost is fat (good) or muscle (bad). If you have lost fat your body fat % will be lower, measurements smaller, and you will look and feel more toned, which is fantastic.

If you have lost muscle (and therefore fat % has gone up, and you look and measure smaller but feel flabbier), are you perhaps following a 'weight loss' plan not a 'fat loss' one? Have you been focussing on calories yet not choosing the right sort of foods? If you have been following the meal plan correctly then is your body under stress, perhaps you're not getting adequate sleep? Are you doing resistance workouts to strengthen and shape muscles rather than steady-state cardio like jogging?

Try keeping a detailed food, exercise and sleep diary and compare it to my recommendations to reveal if you are being truly compliant, and take a look at these pointers:

- **increase protein and fibre** consumption – always the first thing to try

- **lower starchy carbohydrate** intake

- **raise starchy carbohydrate** intake if lowering it doesn't work for you

- increase **exercise** (intensity workouts and gentle walking)

- **reduce steady state cardio** (jogging and power walking) if you're primarily doing this

- address lifestyle issues, in particular **sleep** and **stress**

You have gained fat

Have you lost weight? Losing weight in the form of muscle will show up as an increase in body fat %, and a flabbier, less toned appearance. Are you therefore perhaps following a 'weight loss' (low fat, calorie controlled) plan not a 'fat loss' one? Have you been focussing on calories yet not choosing the right sort of foods? If you have been following the meal plan correctly then is your body under stress? Exercising incorrectly (too much steady state cardio, not enough walking and high intensity workouts), too much coffee, not enough sleep; these things all induce stress hormones which encourage fat storing.

Alternatively, if you have *gained* weight (in this case as fat not muscle) then it is possible that you are eating too many calories, so, while I don't advocate calculating everything exactly, being aware and mindful of the calorie content of foods can go a long way to helping you make educated choices around food.

Try keeping a detailed food, exercise and sleep diary and compare it to our recommendations to reveal if you are really following the advice given.

- **increase protein and fibre** consumption – always the first thing to try

- **lower starchy carbohydrate** intake

- **raise carbohydrate** intake if lowering doesn't work (it is possible to go too low)

- be aware that certain foods may be **catalyst foods** for you and are causing rises in blood sugar and insulin, or are actually making your hunger and cravings worse

- **count your calories** over a few 'typical' days to see if you are eating too much; reduce by around 200 calories/day and eat this way for at least a week before making further adjustments, to see if that's all it takes to get results

You have lost fat

Brilliant! Just what we hoped for! The higher percentage of muscle in relation to fat will mean a more efficient metabolism, and increased fat and calorie burning even at rest. How have you been feeling? If you are not unreasonably hungry, do not crave sugary, fatty, salty and starchy foods, and have sustained and balanced high energy levels then this is fantastic, you're following a sustainable lifestyle that is at the same time burning fat.

If on the other hand these issues have been a struggle, then it's time to get them under control before your willpower runs out:

- **raise protein and fibre** intake

- **raise starch** intake slightly

- check that **catalyst foods** are not making your hunger, energy and cravings worse

- try using **cocoa**, **green** and **black teas**, **fibre supplements**, **vinegar**, natural calorie free **sweeteners**, **coffee** in moderation, stimulating **herbal teas**, and consider **BCAA** supplements

- check that lifestyle issues such as **sleep and stress** are not affecting your hunger, cravings and energy levels

You are hungry, have food cravings and low energy levels

This will not do, regardless of whether you are burning fat or not. You are probably either running on willpower (you may well have lost fat and possibly weight too), in which case what you have been doing may be effective but is unsustainable long term, and will make you bored and miserable, and ultimately give up.

Or alternatively you are not following the programme correctly for your body, so still have all those issues which are leading you to overeat the wrong things, so gain weight and fat – perhaps why you came to me in the first place?

A third option is that stress, lack of sleep, etc. is affecting how you feel. Ultimately, the solution to all three scenarios is pretty much the same. Keep a detailed food, exercise and sleep diary and compare it to my recommendations to reveal if you are really following the advice given.

- **raise protein and fibre** intake

- if there is fat loss, **raise starchy carbohydrate** intake slightly; if there is no change or a gain in body fat, **lower starch** intake slightly

- check that **catalyst foods** are not making your hunger, energy and cravings worse

- try using **cocoa**, **green** and **black teas**, **fibre supplements**, **vinegar**, natural calorie free **sweeteners**, **coffee** in moderation, stimulating **herbal teas**, and consider **BCAA** supplements

- check that lifestyle issues such as **sleep and stress** are not affecting your hunger, cravings and energy levels

You are not hungry, have no cravings and your energy levels are good

That's great as you're feeling good, but how about your body fat percentage and weight?

If body fat percentage and/or measurements have gone down, then fantastic – you're following a sustainable programme that's also getting you results.

If, however, your body fat has gone up or stayed the same, then maybe you need to make some tweaks to make sure you are adapting the programme to your body type. If you are satisfying your hunger and cravings by reaching for the very foods you crave (most likely high in sugar, fat and starch as this is what we are biologically programmed to crave for quick energy fixes when blood sugar gets too low) then you will almost certainly not lose fat and quite possibly gain it.

Keep a diet diary as you may not even be aware of what and how much you are eating throughout the day. Also be aware of how stress may be increasing hunger and cravings while decreasing energy – not enough sleep or going too long between eating will almost certainly have this effect.

- go back over the programme guidelines – eat adequate **protein and vegetables**

- **reduce starchy carbohydrate** intake

- **reduce or raise fat** intake – find your 'sweet spot' that makes you feel satisfied and nourishes your body

- use **pre-emptive eating**; eat before hunger sets in to prevent you from over-compensating later

- **increase exercise** – high intensity workouts and gentle walking

- check that **catalyst foods**, lack of **sleep** and **stress** are not making your hunger and cravings worse and lowering your energy

The metabolism killer, does starvation mode exist?

Your body is smart, it doesn't want to starve to death. What people refer to as 'starvation mode' is technically 'metabolic adaptation', your body's way of preserving energy (storing fat) in anticipation of no food being available. But, no surprise, the less you eat, the less you weigh, and the lower your body fat, the slower your metabolism will be to prevent you from starving. This process is normal and unavoidable, though there are things you can do and not do to keep damage to a minimum:

- don't eat too few calories – just low enough to steadily lose weight if you need to, or adequate to maintain your weight (or gain it if needs be)

- eat plenty of protein to help repair, build and preserve muscle mass, which is very 'metabolically active'; lots of muscle = fast metabolism

- do strength and resistance training including high intensity body weight exercise, again to support muscle strengthening and shaping

- keep stress low – stress hormones can also put the brakes on burning fat

If you have been yo-yo dieting for many years, have been eating too few calories for too long, have high body fat and/or low muscle mass, or are or have been under a lot of stress and think you may have damaged your metabolism, regardless of your weight you may need to do a bit more repair work before you see results. But please don't panic; that's why you bought this book and that's why I'm here; to help you get to where you want to be – hop over to my FREE Facebook Group on www.facebook.com/groups/weightlossandfitnessformums/ and ask me and other members whatever you want – I'd be very surprised if you were the only person with the worries you have, so please reach out for support.

So there you have your troubleshooting guide to personalising your diet to make it work for you. It was Einstein who said the definition of madness is doing the same thing and expecting different results. So try, assess, tweak and repeat; be your body's own detective and figure out what works for you!

N.B. Once again, please seek advice from a qualified individual if planning on taking any supplements, and inform them of any conditions you have or medication taken.

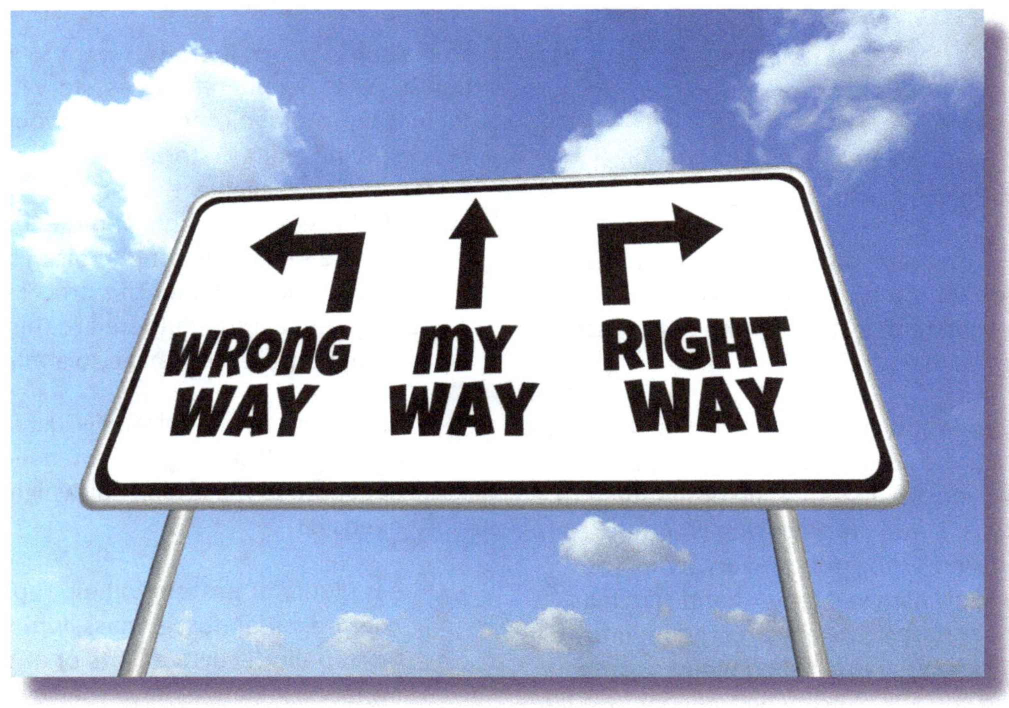

6 LOGICAL (BUT OFTEN MISSED) REASONS YOU'RE OVEREATING – AND HOW TO STOP

If you're overweight or can't lose weight, you're eating too many calories, it's as simple as that. You might even know this already – it's a simple mathematical formula of energy in vs energy out. But the reasons you're overeating could be one or many, so without knowing why you can't stop at less food it's going to be hard to change that.

Note that these six particular reasons for overeating are of the practical, physiological, maths of calories-in calories-out nature. They suggest ways that you may be consuming more calories than you need unintentionally.

If you're overeating for emotional reasons, pay special attention to the previous chapter on mindset and make sure you have the support you need.

Here are 6 common reasons you're overeating and, more importantly, how to stop!

1. You're hungry

This should be pretty obvious, but if your tummy is growling it's going to be very difficult to avoid eating. The trick is to eat a big enough quantity of food without overdoing the calories. If your calorie needs are lower than normal (which they will be if you're trying to lose weight), fill up on plenty of low calorie vegetables, salad and some fruit. Eat plenty of protein – a portion at every meal and snack – as protein is the most satiating macronutrient. Figure out what balance of fats and carbohydrates make you feel best – some people don't feel satisfied without enough carbs, while others are still hungry if they eat a fat-free meal. Choose higher fibre carbohydrates, such as quinoa instead of white rice and oats instead of refined cereals. One of the most filling substances is something called resistant fibre (also known as resistant starch), which is found in green bananas, beans and legumes, and cold, cooked new potatoes or cold cooked rice, so try swapping mashed potato for mashed chickpeas, or use lentil flours to bake with.

2. You're dehydrated

Your body can mistake being thirsty for being hungry, so try having a drink first. Interestingly, warm drinks take longer to leave your stomach than cold ones, so a hot cup of tea or herbal tea might satisfy you more than plain water. If you drink smoothies, make them with less liquid so they're thicker – this makes them slower to digest and more filling. If you eat a low carb diet you might not be holding on to fluids as much, so try adding a little Himalayan salt to filtered water or to your food. Electrolyte drinks are an option, but choose sugar-free ones, unless you're taking part in long distance endurance exercise (such as a run lasting more than 90 minutes) and, for the most part, they're an unnecessary expense. The more protein you eat the more water you need too, since water is involved in the metabolism of protein.

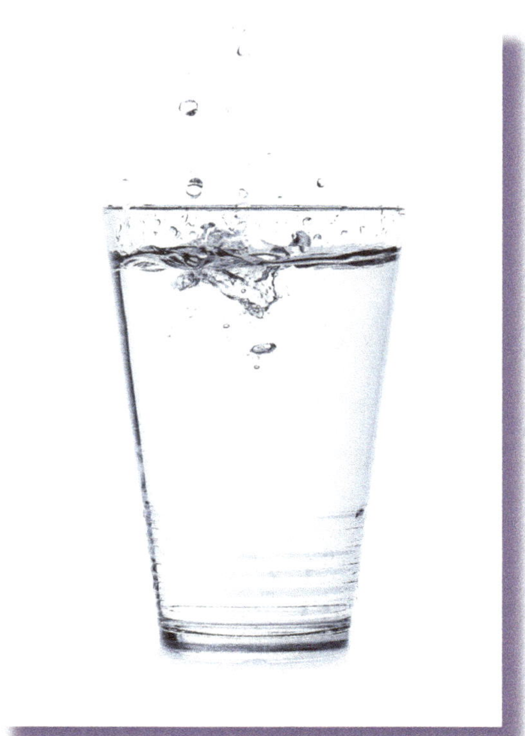

3. You're not paying attention

Mindlessly eating means you won't notice when you're full, so watching TV, checking emails or working could result in eating more from your plate than you really need. If you're really busy and have to work while eating, only put on your plate what you intend to eat. Measure out a portion that's within your calorie and macro requirements and you can happily finish your plate knowing you've not gone over.

4. You eat by the clock

If 4pm is snack time, that's what you'll do. But this is often due to habit rather than actually being hungry. Have you ever been out of routine (perhaps you're in the middle of a meeting you can't get out of) and realised that you got by until an hour later without starving? Try holding off until you're genuinely hungry before eating just because 'it's time'. Similarly, have you ever accepted a chocolate from the tin or piece of someone at work's birthday cake just because it was offered to you? Were you really hungry or just being polite?

5. You eat too often

By this I don't mean you're just eating too much over the day. But rather that if you're eating small amounts often (as opposed to fewer, larger meals) your stomach may not be being stretched enough to fully stimulate a hormone called cholecystokin (CCK), which in turn makes you feel full. Rather than grazing throughout the day try a week of three main meals and see if this reduces hunger and food consumption overall. I say a week, because if your body is used to eating at certain times your appetite will rise at these times out of expectation, so it may take a few days to get used to a new routine.

6. You're not calorie aware

If you're new to dieting and nutrition you simply may not be aware of the nutritional values of foods. Start reading labels, learning about calories, fats, protein and carbohydrates, and consider using an app like MyFitnessPal for a few days to plan and evaluate how much you're actually consuming.

Take a look at your eating habits and see if any of the above could be the reason you're overeating. Can you spot where you've been going wrong? It could be one thing or (more commonly) a combination of a few. Once you figure it out, you can change it.

HOW YOU CAN STOP CRAVING FOOD

The worst thing when you're trying to cut calories and eat less is when you can't stop craving food.

It's not your fault, in fact it's your brain's built-in survival mechanism to ensure you don't die of starvation. Humans began in a time when eating happened whenever you found/caught something edible. Sometimes we ate nothing for days, other times we ate a lot in one sitting. It was unpredictable at best, devastating at worst, and the best thing our brains could do was to make sure we were hungry and searching for food at all times, so that we could fatten up and have 'stores' available for when we weren't able to eat.

Life, thankfully, isn't quite so difficult these days, at least in terms of getting hold of food, and where you can eat a lot on a very low budget in all but the poorest of countries. Food is never far away, and most people have the luxury of never being forced to go hungry.

Only, our brain hasn't cottoned on to this; it still believes we need to eat everything in sight to 'save up' for famine.

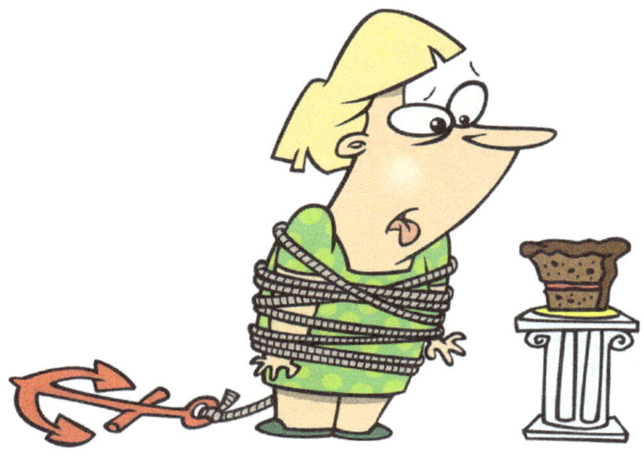

Nowhere else does this mechanism kick in stronger that when we're in a calorie deficit trying to lose weight. That clever primal brain of yours thinks you're being, quite frankly, rather stupid not eating, and will do everything in its power to make you eat, not realising you would actually be healthier if you were a bit slimmer, as it's unlikely that 'famine' will happen.

It all makes for a rather miserable and challenging dieting experience, so how can we 'trick' our brains so that we stop craving food?

10 effective ways to stop craving food

1. **Eat more**
   Yes really! But I mean more volume not more calories. Eat smaller portions of calorific foods and fill up with low calorie vegetables, salad and fruit. You can eat a huge salad with some lean chicken for about the same calories as some 'healthy' snack bars, but a cereal bar doesn't fill you up nearly as much as a large salad.

2. **Eat more fibre**
   Choosing higher fibre options of foods will fill you up more than low fibre ones. Eat the skin on fruit and vegetables where possible, don't drink juices (where the fibre has been removed), and always opt for whole foods and wholegrain varieties that have not been stripped of their fibre during processing.

3. **Eat more protein**
   Protein is the most satiating macronutrient so if you want to keep hunger at bay, eat more of it. As well as meat, fish, eggs and dairy products; swap starches like white rice and mashed potato for higher protein quinoa and mashed chickpeas.

4. **Sleep and relax more**
   When we don't sleep enough our bodies produce more of the hunger hormone ghrelin and less of the 'full' hormone leptin. Stress can be both an appetite suppressant and a stimulant, but most people find their craving for sweet and fatty junk foods increases when they're stressed.

5. **Avoid foods that trigger cravings**
   Though a small selection box chocolate or a teaspoon of peanut butter might not add a lot to your calorie intake, some people find that certain foods are 'once they start they can't stop' foods. Know yours and avoid them until you manage to get a-hold of this all or nothing consumption.

6. **Try certain supplements**
   Try using cocoa, green and black teas, fibre supplements, vinegar (which decreases the GI of a meal), natural calorie-free sweeteners like stevia, coffee in moderation, stimulating or relaxing herbal teas, and consider branched chain amino acid (BCAA) supplements. All these can be useful in combating cravings, but N.B. try the food and dietary strategies first, supplements are always the last strategy to implement in any goal.

7. **Pre-emptive eating**
   Eat before you get too hungry so that you prevent the release of stress hormones to raise blood sugar, and to prevent you from overcompensating later and ultimately eating more overall.

8. **DON'T eat fat free**
   OK, so this goes against the first point of eating larger quantities of lower calorie foods. But adding (or including) fat in a meal is more satisfying than a fat-free meal for most people. Almonds are high in fat yet have been shown to decrease hunger, while many fat-free foods are high in carbohydrates and sugar, which can set off a hunger and craving rollercoaster.

9. **Stick to a schedule**
   Some people feel best on three meals and three snacks a day. Others like two large meals a day. Some people even utilise intermittent fasting and go several hours without eating. Most people do best spreading their daily food intake across 3–6 meals a day, but work out what keeps your hunger to a minimum and helps you personally to stop craving food.

10. **Work out if it's physical or emotional hunger and cravings**
    Genuine hunger starts in the stomach, and responds well to being filled, even if that's low calorie vegetable sticks or even a hot drink. Cravings start in the brain and can be due to feeling low, lonely, angry, bored or any other emotion, even happiness! If you're genuinely hungry you'll eat anything, even a boring plain stick of celery. If you won't try eating vegetables or fruit first, it's probably just a craving.

Whatever you do don't try and stop craving food by willpower alone. You'll cave in eventually and possibly overcompensate by eating way more than you intended. Rather, try the tricks above and see if you can knock those cravings once and for all.

Your daily diary

This next page is a daily diary for you to fill in to keep track of your food and activity levels, of how much you drink and how much sleep you get – all important factors when looking after yourself mentally and physically.

Print off or photocopy seven copies at a time (a week's worth). Hint: set your printer to black and white and draft mode to save ink, and I usually print on to the back of scrap paper too! Or draw a copy or write the information in a notepad.

It's up to you how you go about recording your behaviours, but if you're not where you want to be in terms of your body and health, then you won't know how to improve your behaviours if you don't know what you're currently doing or where you're going wrong. This is where writing it down becomes really useful. These days I don't need to do it so often, but I certainly have in the past.

It's a tactic not just useful for weight loss. When I saw some (rather expensive) private natural health doctors about terrible IBS (that once had me in A&E on morphine) they had me writing down every crumb that passed my lips for weeks. Nobody is ever 100% perfect (I'd argue anyone who is has 'issues'), but I amazed myself how many times I was finishing rejected Weetabix, licking the spoon while baking cakes, and having a bite of pizza. These little things (we're talking a small mouthful) won't add up much in terms of calories, but when you're looking for IBS triggers and food intolerances, that was dairy, wheat and nightshades I was consuming all the time, even when I was supposed to be temporarily cutting them out!

My point is that, as Mums, we are so busy we do things without realising, so by writing it all down it's much easier to see where we're going wrong.

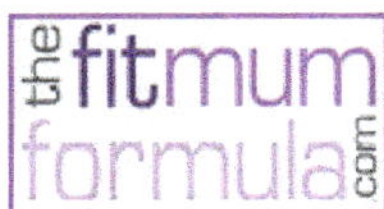

ACTIVITY DIARY FOR ___ / ___ / ___

Food diary

Breakfast	
Lunch	
Dinner	
Snacks	

Exercise diary

| Exercise | Type | | | | | | |
| | Duration | | | | | | |

| Today I walked for: | 15 mins | 30 mins | 45 mins | 60 mins | 75 mins | 190 mins | |

Drinks diary (non-alcoholic drinks consumed today)

| No. | | | | | | | | |
| Type (water/tea): | | | | | | | | |

Sleep diary

| Hours sleep I had last night: | 4 | 5 | 6 | 7 | 8 | 9 | |

HUNGER, FOOD CRAVING AND ENERGY LEVELS DIARY

These three things can literally make or break your long-term success. Willpower is exhaustible. You can only be hungry, put up with craving your favourite treat, or survive on low energy – in other words, getting by on willpower – before it runs out and you are running the risk not just of having a treat (which is fine), but of throwing in the towel and giving up completely. Believe me, I've seen it time and time again.

Honestly, you wouldn't believe how many women I have to persuade to eat more! Fear of gaining weight leads to over-restriction of food and unrealistic exercise plans. And that never works out long term.

Ideally you want hunger to be below 5, food cravings (that's having the craving in the first place, whether or not you actually end up eating the food) under 5, and energy levels above 5.

If your results do NOT fall into these numbers then you need to tweak what you're doing, even if you're losing weight successfully, in order to make your choices a sustainable long-term lifestyle rather than a short-term, short-lived diet. See where to find the information to tweak your programme below.

Print off this chart and complete it every day. At the end of each week compare your hunger, food cravings and energy levels to the changes in your weight, measurements and body fat percentage.

Be a body detective

Do you lose more weight when you are hungrier? Or did eating enough of the right foods to not feel hungry still result in a decrease in weight, or body fat percentage or body measurements, after all?

Did having low energy levels make you more sedentary when you weren't doing a workout, meaning you burnt fewer calories overall and therefore didn't progress as much as you'd have hoped? This is what happens with office workers too. They might be going to the gym every night for an hour, but if they've been sat down, literally, all day, combined with a bad diet this is not going to get results.

What other patterns can you notice? Can you be your very own body detective and use the information about what you ate and did, how you felt, and whether you lost or gained fat to learn how *your* body works best?

Note: Use this space to note down any patterns you see emerging and compare them with your results from the body stats tracker on the next page. Is energy low when hunger is high? Are cravings worse when you are tired?

Week Beginnning (date):

Day/Date	Hunger 1–10	Food cravings 1–10	Energy levels 1–10
Day 1			
Day 2			
Day 3			
Day 4			
Day 5			
Day 6			
Day 7			

Average for the week

To find the average add up all the numbers in one column then divide by 7.

Hunger: ___________________   Food cravings: ___________________   Energy levels: ___________________

BODY STATS PROGRESS TRACKER

Print off this chart and complete once a week. See your body change over time! Allocate a specific day of the week if it helps you remember, for instance every Friday or Monday morning.

Not seeing the results you want? Something needs adjusting.

Check back through this chapter for help with that.

N.B. to avoid confusion choose either imperial (pounds/lb and inches) or metric (kg and cm) measurements for everything but not both.

Body stats tracker chart

Date	Weight	Waist	Thigh	Hips	Upper Arm	Neck	Chest	Wrist	Forearm	Notes:how I feel about my results
Week 1										
Week 2										
Week 3										
Week 4										
Week 5										
Week 6										
Week 7										
Week 8										
Week 9										
Week 10										
Week 11										
Week 12										

MEASUREMENT NOTES

Weight

Weigh yourself first thing in the morning, in light clothing such as underwear, before eating or drinking anything, and after going to the loo. This will ensure your results are as consistent as possible. Scale weight is affected by many things – such as food and drink volume consumed in the last 48 hours (regardless of caloric value), water retention, menstrual cycle, salt and carbohydrate intake, and bowel movements – so we never take the number on the scale as gospel, nor is it necessarily an accurate measure of progress. Muscle is denser than fat, so as you build muscle and burn fat, you may weigh the same (or even more in the case of a slim person wanting to just get fitter and stronger), while being smaller or changing shape. If you have a lot of weight to lose you will most likely lose some if you consistently improve your diet, exercise and lifestyle, and scales can help measure that. But the closer you get to your desired weight the more irrelevant it becomes and you may prefer to stick to other markers of progress.

Waist

The best place to lay the measuring tape is so it crosses through your belly button. Why? Because it doesn't move! Your results will always be consistent and are less likely to be inaccurate due to human error while measuring. It's also pretty much the narrowest part of your waist anyway which is what we are aiming for. Do this measurement first thing in the morning before eating or drinking. Remember, holding fat around your middle isn't the only reason for a larger than desired measurement; having food/drink inside you from consumption during the day (hence I advise measuring first thing), bloating from food intolerances, gas and constipation, can all give you a larger measurement, so take these into consideration if you think you've lost fat from your waist but the tape measurement isn't saying so.

Thigh

Measure the circumference of the widest point of the thigh. Most women complain about their thighs (me too, we all have 'fat' days right?!) but aiming for that coveted 'thigh gap' where the tops of your thighs don't touch when you stand straight, is not only unnecessary, it's stupid.

People come in all different shapes and sizes and someone with the most gorgeously long, lean toned legs might not actually have a 'thigh gap' if they're not built that way.

Hips

Measure the widest point around your hips. This is often lower than people think at first so try checking in a mirror from the front, side and behind to make sure the tape measure is in the right place. If you don't have a lot of weight to lose but would like to firm up your glutes (bottom), exercising the glutes and strengthening them will 'lift' the muscles, giving you a curve and shape you'll be proud to show off in a bikini – but they might ultimately actually measure bigger than before you started The Fit Mum Formula's exercise programme.

Upper arm

Measure round the largest part of the bicep – your upper arm, between your elbow and shoulder. Remember the arms that look good in strappy tops (who doesn't want that?!) aren't the slimmest; you need some muscle there for definition and strength, which will also make daily life easier. If you carry excess weight elsewhere but have slim (but weak) arms you might find this measurement increases as you get stronger.

Neck

Measure at the narrowest point. It might seem odd measuring your neck but it's required for calculating your body fat percentage using the formula below.

Chest

Measure round the widest part of your bust, try not to let the tape sag round your back (you might need someone to help).

Wrist

Measure at the narrowest point. Again, this is required for calculating your body fat percentage using the formula below.

Forearm

Measure at the widest point.

BODY FAT %

The Dexa scan (a bit like an x-ray) is the current gold standard for measuring body fat percentage, followed by hydrostatic (underwater) weighing. Both these have to be done in a facility with the required equipment and resources.

Next are body fat scales, which are used like regular weighing scales (the better ones also have hand grips to hold on to), and skinfold calipers. Scales are easy to use but results vary in accuracy between brands, and even according to variables such as how hydrated you are. Calipers, which 'pinch' various parts of the body and measure how much soft flesh (as opposed to harder muscle, which is more resistant to being pinched), can be pretty accurate if done by someone who knows how to use them correctly. Some personal trainers and dieticians will be able to do this for you, but not all.

For home use the simplest method is with the formula, which for women is:
((Weight(pounds) * 0.732) + 8.987) + (Wrist(inches)/3.14) - (Waist(inches) * 0.157) - (Hips(inches) * 0.249) + (Forearm(inches) * 0.434).

But I don't expect you to do the calculation yourself. At the time of publishing this link to an online calculator was working: http://www.bmi-calculator.net/body-fat-calculator/body-fat-formula.php

If it doesn't work when you try visiting the page (it's not mine), then copy and paste the formula above into a search bar and it should take you to other sites where the calculator can be found.

Note that, as stated before, this is not the most accurate way of measuring body fat % but it is at least something you can get at home as a ballpark number to see where you're currently at and to work on. Rather than seeing it as an exact number, work on creating a trend according to your goals — for most people this will be to see their body fat % getting lower over time.

The American Council on Exercise categorises your results into the following for women:

10%–13% = essential fat

14%–20% = athletic

21%–24% = fit

25%–31% = acceptable

32% + = obese

These are guidelines, as medical definitions of obesity are based on BMI (see below) not body fat percentage. Commonly they tend to correlate; someone who is very heavy will often be carrying a lot of fat. However this isn't always the case, such as with bodybuilders or 'thick set' sporting individuals such as rugby players, who will be heavy but very strong, with more muscle and less fat. At the other end is the 'skinny fat' person who is small (doesn't weigh a lot) but is weak, with not much muscle, so proportionally has a higher percentage of fat.

BODY MASS INDEX (BMI)

The formula for calculating your BMI is:

Weight (kg) ÷ Height (m)^2

For example: 70kg ÷ 1.7m^2 = 70 ÷ 2.89 = 24.2

This 'example' person has a BMI of 24.2

N.B. BMI is not always a great predictor of health. Muscle is denser than fat, and therefore a strong, toned person will weigh more than a weaker, 'softer' person, even if they were the same height and clothes size. Use as a guideline only so you can gauge how your body is changing over time. If you have a lot of weight to lose you will likely lower your BMI, but if you are not significantly overweight and are looking to 'tone up', you may even gain weight by this scale, even though you look better.

Photo results tracker

Print off this photo tracker and stick your photos on to show off your progress!

Take front, side and back photos once a month to assess progress; too often and you may not see results, but seeing your body change over time is so motivating. It's also a better way to track than scales alone, since muscle is dense and will make you 'weigh' more, even if you're actually smaller!

Today's Date: ....

- underwear is best,
  or body-shape revealing sportswear

- try to use the same clothes every time
  you take photos

- you can take pictures by standing in front of a full
  length mirror and photographing the mirror

- alternatively get someone else to take the photos.

Pin your front photo here

Pin your side photo here

Pin your back photo here

Finally, and most importantly, **don't judge yourself**. This is about the journey; it's not about where you are now, it's about where you're going and the progress you're making. Every step forward is a fantastic achievement.

Well Done!

FIXED YET?

If your answer was a resounding NO, then congratulations! You have just realised why a three-week, month, even year-long diet plan will not work.

Why?

Because your body and its needs are always changing. Your nutritional requirements even change daily. Your ability to exercise changes, and not always in a progressive way – you may get injured, or sick, or just feel plain rubbish on occasion. Hungover? Kid been up sick all night? Flu? It happens. And the sooner you learn to accept this and just go with it, the easier life will be.

You don't always have time to make a recipe from scratch. You can't always get to the shops. You will (I hope) be invited to all manner of social, fun, food-centred celebrations, such as meals out, birthdays, Christmas, and even just a catch-up in your favourite coffee shop (or in the soft play zone café, whatever).

You will be presented with 'opportunities' to eat highly calorific and junk food everywhere you go. Vending machines, supermarket offers, the surprise cake your colleague baked you to welcome to back after maternity leave, your mother-in-law's 'eat it or you're not worthy of my son' attitude.

I hope you will try all sorts of physical activities, especially ones that are fun and not just exercise. Wall climbing at your local sports centre, an hour at the trampoline park – heck, I even booked a pole-dancing class with some friends one birthday, and it was the most hilarious night of fun we'd had in ages.

Some days you will be really hungry, others not so much. Some days you will crave chocolate so badly you'll want to scream. In this book I have given you some tools and tactics to deal with this, work out why it's happening, and put action steps in place to reduce the chances of it happening again. It's not always in our control (e.g. a sleepless night due to sick kids), but most of the time, it is totally in your control.

You have the ability, the means and the choices in front of you. I've taught you what, how and why certain tactics work. I've shown you what works for thousands of Mums like you who never believed they had the life, body or mental strength (willpower) to feel and look as good as they'd like to.

They just hadn't figured out yet what worked for them. I invite you to achieve the body, energy, wellbeing and happiness that are possible, by following the steps in this book, and finding out what works for you.

WHAT'S NEXT?

I really hope you enjoyed reading what, I believe, is a book that will change the way you think about food, exercise and your body, for life.

The researchers predict that if the current trend continues, up to 48% of men and 43% of women in the UK could be obese by 2030, adding an additional £1.9–£2 billion per year in medical costs for obesity-related diseases.

If you're reading this, chances are you're one of those already in the overweight or obese categories. But it doesn't have to be this way, and I'm pretty sure you don't want it to be, either.

Just look at all the diets that you've tried, and even the initiatives governments have taken over the years to get us all fit and healthy again. Unfortunately, they're just not working.

Do we continue as we are, doing the same things but more of them? Advising the same diet ideas, experimenting with fads, or researching new drugs to manage the illnesses that arise from poor lifestyle choices (refer to the health timeline in the Introduction for a reminder), and weight loss pills to shed the fat?

Or is it time for a different approach. One that works in harmony with, not against, your body. One that feels natural and instinctive, doesn't give rise to hunger, nutrient deficiencies and a slowed metabolism. An approach that your body was hoping you would be taking from birth, but somewhere along the line you got distracted by misinformation and marketing.

My BodyBack programme takes a different approach to the majority of diet clubs, and even personal trainers. These clubs thrive on you not maintaining results long term. That's why it possibly 'worked' for you in the past, before you put the weight back on and went back to them a second or even third time. I know people who have been on this 'train' for years; they go for their weekly weigh-in like it's the highlight of their week. Sometimes I wonder whether they deliberately don't lose weight because they crave the community and support aspect, and to attend groups they need to be 'heavy enough'. But that's a very big digression that I won't go into here, although having to address such psychological issues does sometimes come into helping my Mum-members, where applicable.

While on the subject, mindset is an important factor to long-term success. So while I'm not really one for asking the Universe to send me a magic unicorn to fix my problems, you've got to have your head pointing in the right direction.

If you think about it, it doesn't matter how awesome the diet and exercise plan is, if your thoughts and feelings aren't aligned with your goals, you won't even stick to the plan, so you won't get results.

Are you ready to dive in and take a different path? If what you've been trying so far hasn't worked, or hasn't worked long-term, then stay on the email list you were added to when you purchased this book (or sign up at thefitmumformula.com) and you'll receive invaluable information that will help you on your journey.

In the meantime, join my free group on Facebook, Weight Loss and Fitness for Mums, where you can reach me any time, chat with other Mums, and get tips and advice on the best way to address your eating, exercise and lifestyle choices.

Or, if you're really serious about committing and making changes for the better, for life, consider becoming one of my BodyBack members, where my Mums not only lose the weight they set out to shed, they also …

- have more energy overall than they have done in years

- have fewer energy dips throughout the day (especially peak-biscuit time, mid-morning and afternoon!)

- sleep deeper, and longer, without it impacting how much they 'get done' during the day

- can survive with cake and biscuits in the house, without eating them all as soon as the need strikes

- eat chocolate! But in a different way, that is good for your body rather than contributing to your problems

- have more energy and focus to spend on work, kids, partners and other interests

- improve self-confidence, so are happier in social situations

- rebalance hormones and energy (as well as improved body confidence), resulting in improved sex drive and love life

- no longer feel ashamed or embarrassed in skimpy clothes on the beach, or feel the need to cover up, even if they're not yet at their ideal weight

- learn to really enjoy food, rather than seeing it as either gluttony or deprivation

- enjoy the taste of treat foods, but no longer crave them or feel like you're missing out if you choose to opt out on occasion

- feel like your old self, like you are doing something for you, rather than being a slave to everyone else

It's all possible if you want it.

ARE YOU READY TO GET YOUR BODYBACK?

Join our community and be supported all the way

We get that life is tough, regardless of whether your kids have flown the nest, you are running your own career, home and everything in between, or even if it's just you and you have little extra funds for babysitters!

When we set about designing this programme, we wanted to make sure it not only 'did what it says on the tin', but that we solved other life issues that generally get in the way of us ladies giving some quality time and care back to ourselves!

You are NOT in this on your own, we really do care and want to be there to help you!

- Online course from the comfort of your home

- Unlimited access 24/7 – work out when it suits you

  - Personal support from me at all times
  - Peer support from other Mum-members

- More cost effective than a gym membership or personal trainer

- 30-minute workouts, no equipment needed

- Online meal plans and cookbook

  - Shape, tone and energise using highly effective techniques
  - Eliminate emotional barriers and improve body confidence

- Guaranteed results – tried and tested on hundreds of Mums

Go to www.thefitmumformula.com
to find out more about how you can get
your BodyBack!

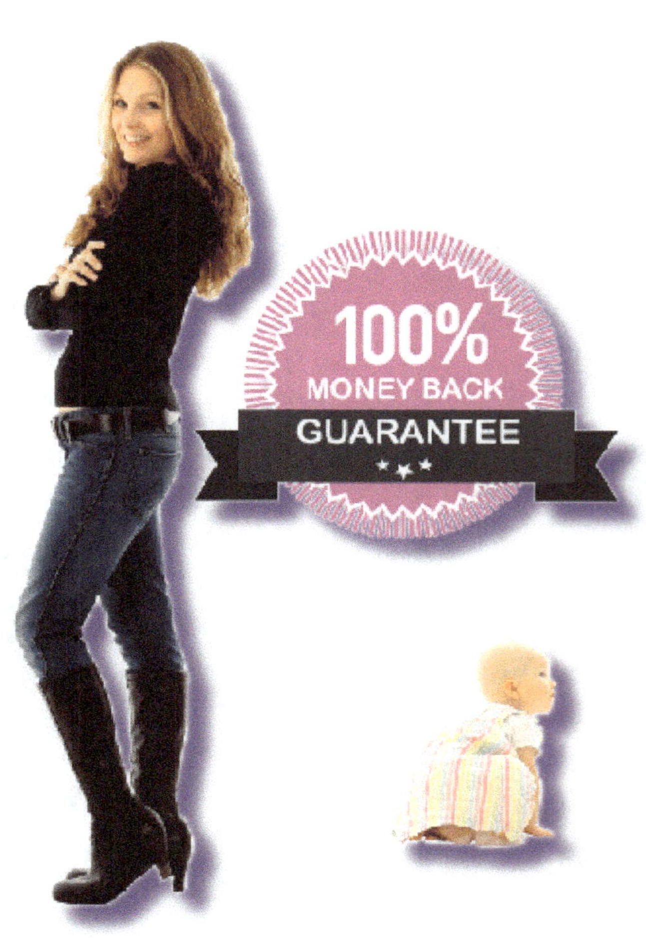

REFERENCES

**These are sites, books and papers that have been referred to or used during the course
 of writing this book.**

http://bmjopen.bmj.com/content

http://onlinelibrary.wiley.com/

http://phys.org/news/2011-06-farming-blame-size-brains.html

http://stateofobesity.org/obesity-rates-trends-overview/

http://visual.ons.gov.uk/how-has-life-expectancy-changed-over-time/

http://www.cancerresearchuk.org/health-professional/cancer-statistics/

http://www.nationalelfservice.net/publication-types/statistics/key-facts-and-trends-in-uk-mental-health-new-fact-sheet-from-the-nhs-confederation/

http://www.nature.com/ajg/journal/v109/n5/abs/ajg201455a.html

http://www.ncbi.nlm.nih.gov

https://en.wikipedia.org/wiki/Decision_fatigue

https://www.acsm.org/docs/brochures/high-intensity-interval-training.pdf

https://www.alzheimers.org.uk

https://www.diabetes.org.uk/About_us/News/diabetes-up-60-per-cent-in-last-decade-/

https://www.noo.org.uk/NOO_about_obesity/adult_obesity/UK_prevalence_and_trends

https://www.sciencedaily.com/releases/2003/12/031204074538.htm

http://terrywahls.com/

Jones DS, Quinn S (eds). Textbook of Functional Medicine. Gig Harbor, Wash.: Institute for Functional Medicine; 2006.

Three Minutes of All-Out Intermittent Exercise per Week Increases Skeletal Muscle Oxidative Capacity and Improves Cardiometabolic Health – http://journals.plos.org/plosone/article?id=10.1371/

Weinstein R. The Stress Effect. New York: Avery-Penguin Group; 2004.

ABOUT THE AUTHOR

Pollyanna Hale has been an ambitious, forward thinking, action taker since the day she was born, never passing by the chance to do something radical or make a huge impact wherever she goes, and she's decided to put that energy toward helping *you*. The years spent in the enclosed shell of a devastating eating disorder were a harsh contrast to the confident, outgoing person she has returned to being today. But that took work. It took many years of self-development, learnt experience and professional help.

Along the journey Polly observed many disturbing trends in how women view, and treat, their bodies. We seem to have moved away from just staying healthy so that we can live and enjoy life, to trying to look as conventionally beautiful as possible. In the process, we've done the opposite; treat foods are viewed as the enemy, yet we eat more junk than ever; exercise as a necessary evil, rather than something that makes us feel good; and clothes sizes as a measure of self-esteem.

It really isn't fair to say 'it's OK for Polly – she's always been slim and has even done modelling work'. If that's your attitude, you must have missed a few pages. This is someone who was sectioned under the Mental Health Act, suicidal and organs failing. Looks mean nothing unless you also feel good, both mentally and physically.

But what doesn't kill you makes you stronger, and it certainly provides wisdom and knowledge you can't acquire without experience, however challenging at the time. Now Polly is passing her lessons on to you.

A qualified Personal Trainer and Nutritionist, Polly has helped hundreds of women, and will help you to look, feel and perform better in your life, be happier for it, and overcome the mental barriers that are stopping you from becoming the person you are both capable of, and deserve to be.

Thank you for reading, I hope you got a lot out of this book. If you need any help, or whatever questions you have, please contact me at any time, Polly. xxx